Glenda

God Bless You Forever

Am so happy to hear your testimony

This is your Turning Point

There so much He needs from you

Enjoy this new journey

Love Always
Cassandra Scott

713.550.5370

DR. CASSANDRA SCOTT

Created 2 Produce
Your Turning Point to Destiny

Copyright © 2012 by Dr. Cassandra Scott
No part of this book may be reproduced, stored in a retrieval system, or transmitted by any means, electronic, mechanical, photocopying, recording, or otherwise, without written permission from the publisher.

Published
by Cassandra Scott Ministries

For ordering
information or special discounts for bulk purposes,
please contact:
Cassandra Scott Ministries
c/o Created 2 Produce
P. O. Box 841236
Pearland, Texas 77584
713.550.3370

www.Created2Produce.com
cscott@Created2Produce.com

Scott, Cassandra
CREATED 2 PRODUCE
2nd edition
ISBN: 978-0-9882936-0-1

Printed in the United States

Created 2 Produce: Your Turning Point to Destiny

TABLE OF CONTENTS

DEDICATION
FOREWORD
ACKNOWLEDGEMENTS
SPECIAL TRIBUTES

CHAPTER 1
The Story   17

CHAPTER 2
Complications   25

CHAPTER 3
Spiritual Difficulties in Conceiving   33

CHAPTER 4
The Process of Waiting   43

CHAPTER 5
Victory   51

CHAPTER 6
Ready, Aim, Fire   61

CONTENTS, CONTINUED

CHAPTER 7
Girl Interrupted 71

CHAPTER 8
Identity Crisis 81

CHAPTER 9
Prepare For A Miracle 95

CHAPTER 10
God's Got This 113

CHAPTER 11
Winning The Battle Of The Mind 131

CHAPTER 12
I Want My Daddy 139

CHAPTER 13
Let It Be 153

DEDICATION

This book is dedicated to my beautiful mother, Naomi Hampton Hilliard. You were truly an example of a woman who was Created 2 Produce. You inspired me with your love and faith. You left to go to your heavenly home on March 5, 2011; but you will never leave our hearts.

You taught me everything I know. You saw my strengths and weaknesses, but it never changed how you believed and loved me. You always put me above yourself, and made me think I could do anything better than anyone. You taught me in spite of what's wrong to hold my head up and keep pushing forward. I miss you so much; I know you are smiling down on me. I remember sitting at your bedside as you were transitioning to heaven. You sang your last song to me, "Jesus build a fence all around me every day," even in your last breath you sent words to protect me forever. I will always love you.

Your legacy lives on through me, my brothers and our children, and the many lives on earth that you have touched.

Your only daughter,
Cassandra Evett (San).

DISCLAIMERS

I would like to make it understood that I am in no way associated with the medical, psychological, or physiological profession. I do not offer the information included in this book as a substitute for professional, legal, medical, mental health, advice or treatment. It is for your general knowledge only. I also do not take responsibility for any individual's marriage or family life, mental or physical health, or illness; nor am I responsible for their healing. I offer no guarantee that anyone will have a stress-free life or that any physical or mental disorder, disease, or illness will be prevented.

I do however, believe that we are spirit beings who have a soul and live in a body according to I Thessalonians 5:23. I also believe that most problems that manifest in a person have a spiritual root, and that Jesus paid the price for our physical, spiritual, and mental well-being (Isaiah 53:5, I Peter 2:24).

During my life, I've been impacted by countless members of the Body of Christ. God knows it is not my intent to omit anyone, offend anyone, or take credit for anyone's work in presenting this book. Any omission of credit is only by mistake. For any such errors, I ask in advance for your forgiveness and support as I endeavor only to represent our Father's love and excellence.

To that end, please enjoy this rendering of CREATED 2 PRODUCE.

Dr. Cassandra Scott

FOREWORD

"The hand of the LORD came upon me and brought me out in the Spirit of the LORD, and set me down in the midst of the valley; and it was full of bones. Then He caused me to pass by them all around, and behold there were very many in the open valley; and indeed they were very dry. And He said to me, "son of man, can these bones live? So I answered, "O Lord God, You Know," Ezekiel 37:1-3

The above passage of Scripture is a favorite of mine, because it epitomizes the concept of life coming from death, victory coming from battle, and growth coming from pain and humiliation. This is the pattern of God over and over again, and it doesn't appear that it is going to change anytime soon. Now, if this premise is true that it will never change, then there must be people that stand up after being knocked down who will give insight to the keys of their victory. We don't need to hear from those who almost went through it, but the voice of experience and overcoming is the prophetic wind that must blow today in our ears; to offer encouragement and witness to the benefit of endurance and faith in God.

Dr. Cassandra Scott is one of these voices who has made it through the storms of life and prevailed. I have watched her in every life circumstance that has come her way and this woman is a fighter and a winner! With a stalwart faith and unbreakable stamina, she has earned the right to prophesy to the bones and this is the time for her voice to be heard.

By sharing her real-life losses, her transparency will leave you with no-excuses for you to quit, turn around and run, or coward out of your battles. With some defeats, and battle-scars, Dr. Scott will give you the how-to on winning in life, relationships, parenting, ministry and life in general. Success is not just spiritual, but it is after the battles in every realm, you see the landscape of your life green and flourishing that you can claim success. After you have fallen, and you get up and begin to ascend to the mountain of your purpose, only then you can claim victory.

Watch how this journey Dr. Scott shares with us will take you through the dark caves of abandonment and aloneness, to the height of achievement and unparalleled anointing and favor with God and man.

Just as with Israel, coming through a series of slumps, and depravation ending up in a valley scattered, disconnected, and without life and finally coming to the place of productivity, life and strength; you will see God's faithfulness over your life as this very precious Handmaiden of the Lord gives us a glimpse of all it takes to die and then live again.

Let every reader, read with expectation, cry with hope, and be astonished at the level and depth of suffering Dr. Scott has endured, and then be prepared to rejoice, shout and dance when you see the outcome of her pain; now a Mighty Battle Ax for God, strong in faith, prayer and power that is making an impact on her generation in social, political, practical and spiritual spheres.

Now, get ready to see your suffering and experiences differently; not to do you harm or evil, but to bring you to your purpose and your assignment. Accept the God given reason for it all. Here's the good news: "We all were created to produce and your bones will live again!"

The Most Reverend (Dr.) Corletta J. Vaughn
Presiding Prelate: Go Tell It Ministry Worldwide, Inc.
Detroit, Michigan

ACKNOWLEDGEMENTS

I stand amazed at God's goodness and His grace. I never would have made it this far without the power of God. God has been with me every step of the way. I will serve Him for the rest of my days. I thank Him for the favor and provision that He provides. How could I know that I was Created 2 Produce without His word and presence? I could not have made it through all the challenges and surely wouldn't have been able to write this book. My desire is to please Him in all that I say and do. To God Be The Glory!

To my children – Garelyn Evett, Gabrielle Chrishelle and Gary Emerson II. What gifts you are from God! The doctors said I would never be able to have any children but God and his mercy and grace gifted me with each of you. I love you all with all my heart. I love the relationship we all have and all the times we spend special time with each other. We have been through so much but I believe it was training for the journey ahead. I admire your resilience and determination to press past every obstacle and keep moving forward. You have supported me in all I say and do. I decree and declare that all your needs shall be met and you will walk in Heaven's best!

To my father – Edwin H. Hilliard. You always told me to never give up and keep my relationship with God the center of my life. Your words of encouragement and prayers have lifted me beyond words that I could ever write on paper. I am so happy that God choose you to be my father. I will always cherish the wisdom you impart into my life.

To my brothers – Kennith and Roscoe. You are the best brothers in the whole wide world. God knew I needed to be born between the two of you. You have covered me. You have sacrificed and stood in the gap for me all of my life. What would I have done without the two of you? I love you with all my heart and soul. Thank you for believing in me.

To my niece – Kennisha Charles. You are the greatest. Your warm smile and continued support have pushed me beyond my wildest dreams. You have been with me since you were born. Thank you for always standing by my side. Your mom and dad let me practice taking care of you before I had any children of my own. I love you and cherish you for being a solid rock in our family.

Doris Grace Scott – You taught me how to be a first lady. You prayed for me, spoke wisdom to me, loved me and told me how proud you were to be my mother in law – I will remember you all the days of my life – I miss you so much – absent from the body, present with the Lord. I know you are smiling at me from Heaven.

Bishop David M. and Pastor Claudette Copeland. Thank you for your continued love, support and prayers. You have been an amazing spiritual covering for me and the members of Turning Point Faith Ministries.

Apostle Corletta Vaughn. Thank you for being my spiritual mother. Interceding, mentoring, coaching and directing me. You pointed me like an arrow in the right direction. You made me focus. I am eternally grateful. Thank you for asking me to consider in my pain, *"What's Next?"*

To my friend for life – Veronica Harrison. Thank you for covering me in prayer and helping me push through producing this project. You have been with me since pre-kindergarten. Always looking over my shoulder to make sure I had all of my I's dotted and my T's crossed. God knew I needed you then and now. Your sacrifice will never be forgotten.

To my friend and leadership development coach, Merle E. Ray. Where would I be without you? Even when I thought I could not go forward, Merle was there at the beginning of my turning points to coach me and help me develop as a leader, and enhance my God-given talents.

Gloria Archie, Martha Hardin, Pastor Eleanor Murray, Stephanie Glynn, Michelle Baines, Cynthia McConathy, Tongela Clark, Carol Smith, Dorthy Fields, Dorothy Leonard, Pastor Liddie Owens,

ACKNOWLEDGEMENTS

Apostle Jacqueline Phelps, and Stephanie King – Thank you for your intercession. You were spiritual midwives. When I wanted to give up and couldn't even pray or see my way you helped me to press thru until I could see that I was Created 2 Produce. Thank you for never giving up on me.

Turning Point Faith Ministries – Thank you for your love and support. I love each of you with all of my heart. You shall empower kingdom growth in faith, families, finances and futures. You will trust God and live destiny. I am so glad that God gave you to me and me to you – for such a time as this! You are a special gift from God. I am honored to be your pastor. God has an incredible plan for each of you and our church.

CSM Directors, Prayer line and Bishop Frank Rush. What a team of intercessors. God knew I needed each of you. In May of 2010, I obeyed God and started the 6am prayer line. WOW I didn't know that all of you would be in that simple act of obedience. I kicked and screamed wondering why I needed to start a prayer line. I am so glad I did. I would have missed the open door to be blessed with such a beautiful team of intercessors. Prayer is the key, faith unlocks the door. What a privilege it is to pray with you on a daily basis. God put you in my life to show me his power and glory. I stand amazed at all that has been birthed because our paths crossed by the divine plan of God. No one could have put this together but God. I stand amazed. There is a blessing in the cluster.

I thank the Lord for the many men and women of God who spoke into my life and gave me hope and encouragement along the way to be the woman of God that I am. I want to give special thanks to Bishop G. Emerson Scott, Pastor Connie Brooks, Merle Ray, Bishop Ira and Pastor Bridget Hilliard, Pastor Samuel H. Smith, Alyce Kinney, and Pastor Floyd and Beatrice Young.

SPECIAL TRIBUTES

To *my wonderful mother, pastor, friend and teacher:* First, I want to say that I am so proud of your accomplishment in writing your first book. This is just one of the many accomplishments of your turning point. I can't imagine the places that God will take you from this moment on. You have been a true inspiration in my life and to others. Because of everything that you have poured out, you will not have room enough to receive what God will pour back into you. I look forward to your bright future with many trips and vacations, just don't forget me along the way!

**Your first favorite child,
Garelyn Evett Scott**

To My Superwoman:

God is not through with you yet. As you begin this next journey, be prepared for all the mind-blowing blessings that God has for you. I love you with all of my heart and I thank you for all of the sacrifices you have made; not only for your family, but for the Body of Christ as well! Continue to listen to the voice of God, and remember not to get too comfortable, because God is going to move you to the next level at any moment. You mean the absolute world to me and nothing could ever replace a mother's love!

**Love your favorite child,
Gabrielle Chrishelle Scott**

I love you mom you are very encouraging to me. You always lead me in the right direction and keep me on track. You keep me focused on what I have to do to be successful in life. When I feel like I'm down and out, you teach me how to have faith in God. I am so proud that God gave you to me as a mother, and a spiritual teacher. I know that you are always there for me. Congratulations on writing your first book; Created 2 Produce!

**Love your only son and your favorite child,
Gary Emerson Scott II**

1
The Story

Growing up, I often spent days staring out of my tiny bedroom window and dreaming about my future. With gospel great Aretha Franklin singing *Amazing Grace* or *Sacred Secrets* in the background, I spent hours listening to music and praising God with excitement in my heart. As young as age 12, I can remember having visitations from God. I remember one time a strong light flooded my room and I began to cry as I continued to lift His name.

My bedroom was the middle room in a three-bedroom house with one bathroom, a kitchen and garage. I preferred to spend my time in there. I felt safe there. It was the one place where I felt as though I could escape the world around me. Even though my mom would often try to lure me out, I preferred dreaming, pretending and being alone. Sometimes Mom would say, "San, come out of that room. Sit here and let's talk while we do our nails and feet." But I rarely accepted her invitation. I think I wanted to spend so much time alone because I was ashamed of my family's pitiable existence and I felt as though I never really fit in anywhere. So I secretly dreamed big dreams of someday escaping that tiny bedroom that was only big enough to fit a twin size bed, small dresser and closet; that closet was not even large enough to sneeze in. I often thought, *One day I want to be married, have children, a car, own a home, and live happily ever after.*

Many people called me an introvert. However, when it came to proclaiming the Good News, I was anything but. I remember one occasion when I was in the in 6th grade, my teacher asked me to come up and lead the class in the Pledge of Allegiance and Prayer. I remember doing what she said and suddenly ended up shouting, *"Repent, the kingdom of God was at hand!"* I told them that God was on his way back and if they were not saved, they needed to get saved today. It was so funny; the boys that used to chase us with frogs everyday began asking "What must I do to be saved?" They began asking me, *"Is He coming today?"*

My parents named me Cassandra. Growing up, I had no idea how much my name would foretell my future. The name "Cassandra" is of Greek origin. It means "helper of mankind." In 2010, it ranked 328 out of the top 1000 most popular girls' names in the United States. Although I knew what my name meant and that names often declare one's destiny, I challenged myself thinking, *What can I do to help mankind, when I don't even have enough to help myself?* My vision was blurred; my resources were limited, and—at least in my eyes—all odds were against me.

My parents—Edwin and Naomi Hilliard —didn't have much. Growing up in Houston, Texas in the inner-city neighborhood of Kashmere Gardens, I often questioned whether anything good could ever come out of there. I equated who I was with my circumstances. For example, one day My mom said,

"Take this grocery list and these food stamps and make groceries for me." I agreed, but in my mind I was so ashamed of having to pay for my items with food stamps.

When I went with my friends, they had real money - not food stamps. I remember going in the store and looking down every isle before looking at the shopping list, to make sure I didn't see anyone that I knew. Sometimes I spent hours in the store because as soon as I got ready to approach the lane to pay, I saw someone else that I knew.

We didn't have a car; we rode public transportation - *Metro*, Yellow cab, or my mom would get someone to take us wherever we had to go. It was hard for my mom, but you better know she got us where we needed to go. One Easter Sunday morning, our ride didn't come to pick us up. Mom called Yellow cab. *Oh my God,* I thought. *It's bad enough we have to go in a cab, but its yellow and everyone will see it!* Rest assured, when we got to church in Forth Ward, Texas, all the kids were standing outside and saw us. I could have melted! I wanted to disappear regardless of how sharply dressed we were! I remember watching and hearing the kids point and laugh at us as we pulled up. I was crushed.

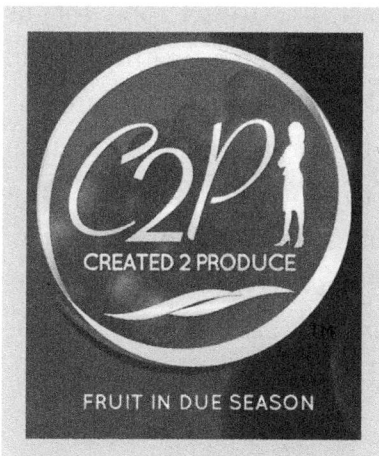

God was calling me in the midst of the cards I had been dealt.

My mom and dad were separated, but to me, they were both great parents, and I loved them both so much. Although they had problems they couldn't work through, my brothers and I always felt loved. I thought: *Why can't my family be together? We are believers.* I was embarrassed that my family was separated. I watched my friends climb up on their dad's lap, kiss and hug him, and talk about their day. I longed to do the same thing. I would walk slowly and observe, longing for every moment of that. I remember our next door neighbors, the McGowan's on one side and the Flagg's on the other. I admired them so much and they were just like family to us.

I am reminded of a man named Gideon who was called, "a mighty man of valor." Gideon also had challenges equating his identity with his circumstance. His task was to get food for his family, even though hostile invaders made growing, gathering and preparing the food almost impossible. Gideon was resourceful. He put a winepress to double duty by turning it into a sunken threshing floor. It lacked ventilation to blow the chaff away, but at least it was hidden from his enemies, the Midianites. When people referred to Gideon as that "mighty man of valor," he must have thought *do you know my status? My family is of the least; you must have the wrong address.* Although he had limited visionary abilities, Gideon was still committed.

Gideon was working in his threshing floor when God sent him a message with a challenge. Gideon was surprised when God told him to go in the strength he had and save Israel from the hand of the Midians. Gideon didn't want to jump into a task that he was ill-prepared to do. In order to convince Gideon that he was equipped for the call on his life, the Angel of the Lord had to overcome three objectives Gideon had:

✓ (1) Gideon's feelings of responsibility to his family's welfare,

✓ (2) His doubts about his calling and

✓ (3) His feeling of inadequacy for the job.

Once Gideon was convinced of his call, he obeyed with zest, resourcefulness, and speed. He dedicated those personality traits to God, with whom he was now personally acquainted. Through Gideon's story, I realize that growing up, God was calling me in the midst of the cards I had been dealt.

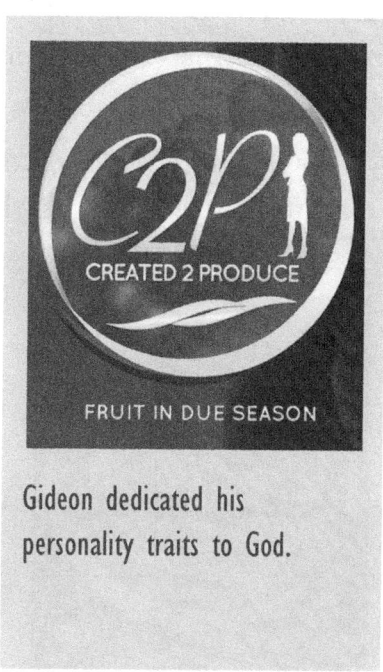

Gideon dedicated his personality traits to God.

I was called to get food for my family. I was created to produce. That food is the Word of God and I was called to grow, gather, and prepare men and women to reach their turning points in life. It surprised me that God would want to use me. I felt, and I still feel unprepared at times. The feeling of inadequacy tormented me day and night when I was a little girl. I never thought I would or even could soar. People made me nervous, especially the loud talking people who had a Word and talked nonstop.

But now I dedicate my personality traits to God. These traits do not define who I am. His Word does. Gideon had his weak moments and failures, but he was still God's servant. If you can see yourself in Gideon's weakness, can you see yourself in Gideon's strength? His strength was he was willing to serve! Remember, Gideon was a man who obeyed God by giving his full attention to the task at hand. <u>Give your full attention to God and believe that He will prepare you for tomorrow when</u> it comes.

Once I grew older, I faced a new more haunting problem. I had menstrual cycles maybe twice a year. Early on, I knew something wasn't right. The doctor told me that I did not ovulate, or produce eggs from my ovaries. In other words, she was telling me I couldn't have children. I was crushed. I remember going to the hospital with my family to visit with people from our neighborhood and church that were sick. I couldn't go to the hospital without going by the nursery floor to see all of those beautiful babies. Oh how I wanted a child of my own someday! I prayed that I would meet someone without children because I wanted to share that experience with the man that I loved, but my womb was shut.

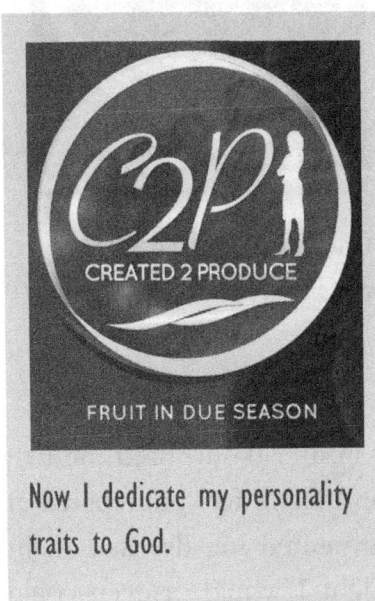

Now I dedicate my personality traits to God.

THE STORY

I prayed and prayed asking God for a breakthrough in this area. It seemed as if nothing was happening. I'm reminded of Hannah in the Bible. Like me, all she wanted was a baby. But God had other plans - bigger and better plans. I didn't realize it then, but my wants didn't compare to the vision God really had regarding me. My doctor put me on medication to help me ovulate; she told me to call the office every morning before I put one foot on the floor.

I had to take my temperature everyday and call the results in to the nurses so they could track my results. If my temperature rose, the nurse said I was to have intercourse because my chances to conceive were greater. This went on for about 2 years; I was drained and it wasn't fun anymore. Trying to make a baby was like having a job. I got to the point where I said, *"Forget it; I don't want to have a baby. This is just not for me."* A month went by and my temperature stayed high. This meant that pregnancy was a strong possibility. My temperature rose and never came down. I went to the doctor and they announced, *"You are pregnant!"* I was so happy I didn't know what to do.

My joy, however, was short lived. Within a couple of weeks, I started spotting, and before I knew it, I'd had a miscarriage. I was devastated and fell into a deep depression. I thought, *What kind of God am I serving?*

My turning point was one Sunday morning as I sat in the balcony fighting within myself about going up to the altar. As I struggled to get up, the enemy reminded me that I had a run in my stockings and I should not move. Somewhere in the midst of that struggle and with tears running down my eyes, I found myself in front of the church giving my life to Christ. Then, God connected me with this powerful woman of God, Cassandra Scott, an amazing woman who pushed me out of the boat and into my purpose. My life has not been the same, since that great day. I have had many turning points in my life. I am now a Co-pastor in the body of Christ, a prayer line visionary, entrepreneur, and a better wife, and mother. I give God all the honor and the glory for my turning points.

Pastor Shiewanda Nelson

2

Complications

I learned so much that I never knew about getting pregnant. In this chapter I want to share with you what I learned about my personal complications and how they related to my physical experience as well as what I have now learned about my spiritual experiences. It is my hope that by sharing my experiences and knowledge gained here, you may find the courage and strength to overcome yours. I caution you again though that every woman is different and this is just my personal experience; you should not look at this as medical advice, but seek the attention and expertise of your medical provider for your own particular situation.

Before I had children, I often asked myself, *What is wrong with me?* It seemed all throughout my life everything was such a struggle. By the time I was married, I wanted a break from the continual flow of difficulties. I desperately wanted to experience a continual flow of blessings instead of constant struggle. I wanted to bear children.

Consider the word, "complication." It's both a noun and a verb that means: *1. the act of complicating; 2. a complicated or involved state or condition; 3. a complex combination of elements or things; 4.*

something that introduces, usually unexpectedly, some difficulty, problem, change, etc. A sample sentence using the word, complication, might sound something like this: *Because of the complications involved in traveling during the strike, we decided to postpone our trip.*

Well "complications" were staring me right in my face! Since my body refused to ovulate, in 1987, my doctor informed me of the complications and what I'd need to do in order for me to get pregnant, Before I became knowledgeable on the complications, I was a wreck!

I remember being in a store and a lady I knew was there; when I went up to speak to her, she just looked at me as if she didn't know me. I said, *"I'm Cassandra Hilliard Scott."*

She replied, *"I didn't know who you were, Are you pregnant?"* I said, *"No."* I tried to smile, but I was sinking inside thinking: *Why is it that can't I get pregnant, yet I look pregnant? What is wrong with me?* I continued to wonder: *Why am I gaining so much weight?*

When I went to my doctor for my yearly exam, I asked her why was I gaining so much weight and looking pregnant. Was I pregnant? And of course, I wasn't – and I was not having a monthly cycle either! This was all so confusing to me; I asked, *"What in the world is wrong?"* The doctor diagnosed me; she said, *"Your body doesn't ovulate."* She explained that I would have to do two things: 1) endure a procedure known to counteract *"Anovulation"* though a fertility drug called, *clomid,* and 2) learn to monitor my – *"basal body temperature"* and be at peace.

How can I do all that? I wondered. *What does all this mean? And what about these new terms my doctor's throwing at me: "Anovulation?" and "Basal Body Temperature?"*

Anovulation

I learned that anovulation means lack of ovulation or absent ovulation. Ovulation, which is the release of an egg from the ovary, must happen in order to achieve pregnancy. If ovulation is irregular, but not completely absent, this is called oligovulation. Both anovulation and oligovulation are kinds of ovulatory dysfunction. Ovulatory dysfunction is a common cause of female infertility, occurring in up to 40% of infertile women.

I further learned some things about how anovulation and ovulatory dysfunction cause infertility. For a couple without infertility, the chances of conception are about 25% each month; so even when ovulation happens, a couple isn't guaranteed to conceive. When a woman is anovulatory, she can't get pregnant because there is no egg to be fertilized. If a woman has irregular ovulation, she has fewer chances to conceive since she ovulates less frequently. Plus, it seems that late ovulation doesn't produce the best quality eggs, which may also make fertilization less likely. Also, it's important to remember that irregular ovulation means the hormones in the woman's body aren't quite right. These hormonal irregularities can sometimes lead to other issues like lack of fertile cervical mucus, thinner or over-thickening of the endometrium (where the fertilized egg needs to implant), abnormally low levels of a necessary hormone - progesterone, and a shorter luteal phase – which is important when a couple is trying to get pregnant.

I asked, *"Is this something that can be cured?"* My doctor gave me the run-down. She started by suggesting a medicine called clomid because I didn't have a monthly cycle. My doctor said, *"Clomid is the most well-known fertility drug. About 25% of female factor infertility involves a problem with ovulation, and clomid, as a fertility drug, is easy to use (taken as a pill, not an injection), with not too many side effects.* She continued, *It's pretty inexpensive compared to other fertility drugs, but is effective in stimulating ovulation 80% of the time.* I continued to listen to my doctor, and after taking all of what she said into my thinking, I said, *"I'm going to strive to do all I'm hearing, and believe God for a miracle".* The complications of conceiving were tormenting my mind. I dreamed about it while I slept; I thought about it while awake. I would be talking to people, thinking about children as they were talking! Everything became such a chore. I needed to relax and just enjoy life, but I was so consumed with becoming pregnant. I couldn't sleep, eat or be happy; I was consumed with having a child. I woke up every morning wondering if this would be the day that I would conceive. All I wanted was to have a child. I was happy and sad when I saw other women with children. It was normal to have kids, so why wasn't I normal? My womb was closed!

Basal Body Temperature

Basal body temperature (BBT) is the temperature of your body at rest. I learned that taking your temperature first thing in the morning, before you get out of bed, eat, drink or go to the bathroom, will give you the most accurate basal body temperature. So every morning before getting out of bed, I had to reach over, take my temperature, and put it on a monthly

Complications

chart. When charting your BBT, I was told to purchase a special thermometer called a BBT thermometer. It records temperatures to the tenth degree and is the most precise thermometer on the market. By charting my temperatures, I learned to see patterns in my menstrual cycle, with the hopes of being able to determine when I was ovulating. My doctor told me it was important for me to learn the dos and don'ts of taking my basal body temperature, so I stayed on top of it. I became fully equipped with charts and graphs and followed every instruction.

Fertility charting is a great way for women to take control of their fertility. In this process, I learned how to use a graph paper chart to plot my body basal temperature and prepare for the right time to conceive. You can find sample charts to download and use by doing a search on the Internet for body basal temperature charts. Here are some vital insights I received from going through this process.

During the first part of a woman's menstrual cycle, basal body temperatures will be lower. The first half of your menstrual cycle is called the "follicular phase." Just before ovulation, you will have a slight drop in temperature followed by a sharp rise in temperature. Not all women will have a drop in temperature before ovulation but if you notice your temperature drop, you should start having intercourse then. Around the time of ovulation, you will see a rise in temperature. By the time you notice this rise in temperature, you have already ovulated. That is why charting works best when done for a few months. What you are looking for is a rise in temperature of about .4 degrees or more after ovulation. If you have ovulated your temperature will remain higher. If your temperature remains higher for three days or more, then you can assume you have ovulated. But be sure to check with your doctor.

To God is the Glory for the things He has done, for He has done great things, whereof we are glad.

Pastor Cassandra, I thank you for allowing me the opportunity to serve you as your Executive Administrator fifteen years ago. I will for be forever grateful to you for seeing something in me that I did not see in myself. From day one I was drawn to serve you, in obedience to God, in serving you came many benefits. As I watched you serve God, I was able to pattern the art of servitude. Though serving you, I have matured in wisdom and have developed those hidden gifts and talents that in this season, I am able to serve with a spirit of excellence.

God Bless you and I love you. For you were created to produce great men and women of God.

Mack R. Lee, Elder

3

Spiritual Difficulties in Conceiving

In order to find the peace that my doctor suggested, I needed examples of women in the bible that had the same complications as I did. When I started researching, my mouth dropped. The Bible says, "There is nothing new under the sun." Nothing was really wrong with me. I had reached a turning point that God would use so I could help others birth the blessings of the Lord in the earth at His appointed time.

Just to name a few... Sarah (Isaac), it took 25 years, Rebecca (Jacob & Esau), it took twenty years, Rachel (Joseph), Hannah (Samuel), Elizabeth (John the Baptist). There are many stories of women in the Bible who struggled with infertility and the pain of not having children.

The Bible not only shares the stories of these "barren women," but also offers hope and comfort during these times. God indeed is the creator of life, and the God of comfort and peace.

Are there areas in your life that are barren? Below are scripture references that I quoted and found hope in during my years of what seemed to be "barrenness." To those who may consider themselves "barren" today, the Bible says, "neither male nor female will be barren." Be encouraged in whatever stage of the journey you are in. I encourage you to pray God's Word and speak blessings into your life on a daily basis.

Scriptures of Hope

Children are a blessing from God:

Psalm 113:9 He gives the barren woman (Cassandra) a home, making her (Cassandra) the joyous mother of children. Praise the LORD!

Psalm 127:3-5

Behold, children are a heritage from the LORD, the fruit of the womb a reward. Like arrows in the hand of a warrior are the children of one's youth. Blessed is the man who fills his quiver with them! He shall not be put to shame when he speaks with his enemies in the gate.

Psalm 139:13-16

For you formed my inward parts; you knitted me together in my mother's womb. I praise you, for I am fearfully and wonderfully made. Wonderful are your works; my soul knows it very well. My frame was not hidden from you, when I was being made in secret, intricately woven in the depths of the earth. Your eyes saw my unformed substance; in your book were written, every one of them, the days that were formed for me, when as yet there was none of them.

John 16:21

When a woman (Cassandra) is giving birth, she has sorrow because her hour has come, but when she (Cassandra) has delivered the baby, she (Cassandra) no longer remembers the anguish, for joy that a human being has been born into the world.

James 1:17

Every good gift and every perfect gift is from above, coming down from the Father of lights with whom there is no variation or shadow due to change.

Psalms 56:9

The day that I (Cassandra) pray, the tide of the battle turns!

In addition to those Scriptures, I want to share some ways to cope with your difficulties. As I saw babies, babies, and more babies around me, it was hard to imagine that anyone could even begin to relate to what I was going through. Never in my life had I seen so many babies. It's so <u>important to find someone to talk to; and yes, there are times you should talk to your husband about it. But, I also found many times, my husband needed a break from all the "why can't we have a baby" talk. Therefore, I think another woman can better understand how your identity, as a woman, can feel so tied to the ability to bear children.</u> Before you seek someone out, I strongly encourage you to ask God first, "Who it should be?" Ask Him to show you someone who is sensitive enough to really listen, and mature enough in their faith, to help you see Him through your pain and slowly move beyond it.

Eventually, I found some mature Christian friends whom I could talk to amidst my struggle. Some of them had experienced challenges that were similar to mine. Others had several children, and were simply understanding and extremely helpful. While in the waiting process, I would consider starting a Bible study/support group. This will help you while you help others in the process. Getting together with other women in similar situations, sharing our struggles, and studying God's Word with the purpose of spiritual growth is a tremendous time of healing.

Spiritual Wisdom

1. **Don't neglect time in God's Word.** As you long for a child, it's easy to start to blame God; I know I did. I was angry with him for the process. I didn't even want to pray sometimes, I had to confess my sin and ask Him to cleanse me and heal me from all unrighteousness. I often thought, *He's the Creator of life, after all, so why doesn't He create a life within me?* As I forgave Him, the time was drawing near!

Even if you feel this way, don't stop spending time with Him through reading His Word and prayer. Tell Him how you're feeling. He can take it, and best of all, He understands. Search the Bible for words of comfort (the Psalms is the place where I often went), for wisdom, for understanding, for faith to trust Him. Different women need to learn different things through their infertility journey. Maybe it's you inability to understand the character of God, to know without a doubt that He never changes, that He's good no matter what. Maybe, like me, you need to understand that God's gift of children is not about

Spiritual Difficulties in Conceiving

whether you deserve it or not. God gives different blessings to different people, and I wasn't able to enjoy the blessings He had given me, because I was too consumed with looking at the blessing of children in other people's lives and thinking, "*Now why didn't He give me that?*" I think Jesus outlines that principle for us in the parable of the workers in Matthew 20:1–16. <u>God does with His favor what He pleases. It's not about who we think deserves it or what we think is fair.</u> As my mother in the spirit said, "<u>The distribution of God's favor depends completely on His sovereign grace and does not conform to human expectations or norms.</u>" It's all about the redeeming power of God. ✱ *AMEN*

2. Get your focus off of yourself. One pitfall of infertility (and any form of suffering for that matter) that I fell into was focusing on me and my own pain. All I could think about was my struggle, my hurt, my problem. But God led me out of that narrow viewpoint to remind me that every single person here on earth has some sort of pain or suffering they've gone through, are going through, or will go through, in the future. In fact, my infertility now seems like a small thing compared to the other challenges I have had since then, and that others I know have experienced. By taking my focus off myself, I was also able to see the ways God had blessed me and to be grateful

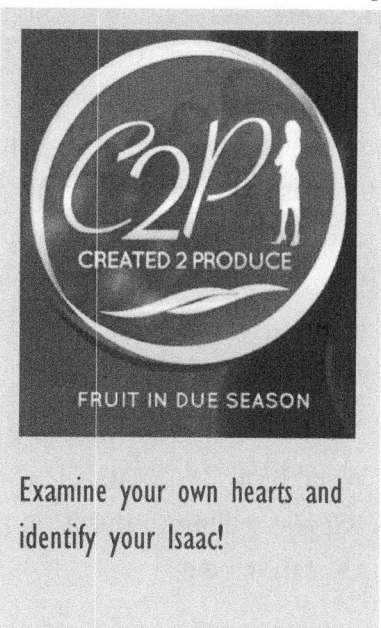

Examine your own hearts and identify your Isaac!

to Him. Eventually, I was also able to "give thanks in all circumstances" (1 Thess. 5:18), even the circumstance of infertility. I wasn't necessarily thankful *for* my infertility, but I was thankful God was walking beside me through all the ups and downs, and for how He changed me in the process. And as I've shared my story with others, I've been thankful for some strengthened family relationships and opportunities to encourage other women who are going through the same struggles.

3. **Surrender your desires to God.** Probably the most important thing you can do in the midst of infertility is to surrender your hopes, your desires, and your future to God. That's easier said than done, I know. I clenched my fingers around wanting to have a child for a very long time. Can you imagine, once God blesses you with what you so long desired; then one day, I heard the story of Abraham in Genesis 22, when God asked him to sacrifice that long-awaited gift of a son. As I read the Scripture, I thought how insensitive, that God would give you something and then ask you to sacrifice it. Don't let me go into what I know God has given me, and it had to be sacrificed?

I challenge you to examine your own hearts and identify your "Isaac." What is it that you love more than anything else? Are you willing to put it on the altar and say, "God, if you want it, you can have it?"

I finally told God that one day and I meant if from the bottom of my heart. I prayed, "God if it is not your will for me to conceive, I leave this sacrifice on the altar and I don't want it if you don't want it. Bathed in tears, I realized that morning that knowing my desire for children was Number One in my life, not my relationship with God. I knew that surrendering this desire didn't mean God would automatically cause me to get pregnant (which He didn't) or that the struggle would completely go away (it didn't either). But what I did find was peace; the peace of knowing God was in control of my life no matter what He did or did not bless me with. In fact, I was able to echo the words of David in Psalm 16: "LORD, you have assigned me my portion and my cup; you have made my lot secure. The boundary lines have fallen for me in pleasant places; surely I have a delightful inheritance (vv. 5–6).

My turning point lessons:

- I grew and was strengthened in my faith - Abraham is a great example of faith in the Bible, and his biggest test of faith was believing God for a child. Hebrews 11:11-12 tells us *"By faith Abraham, even though he was past age—and Sarah herself was barren—was enabled to become a father because he considered him faithful who had made the promise. And so from this one man, and he as good as dead, came descendants as numerous as the stars in the sky and as countless as the sand on the seashore."*

- I developed patience and character. When we accept Christ in our lives and decide to live for Him, it doesn't mean the rest of our lives will be on easy street. The Bible guarantees us that we will have trials and difficulties to deal with in life. Thankfully, God also gives us a promise that all our difficulties will ultimately end in our good if we keep seeking Him (Rom 8:28).

- God showed me my true source of joy. Most Christians are familiar with Psalm 37:4 *"Delight yourself in the LORD and he will give you the desires of your heart."* This is a great scripture to meditate on and remember, but many people seem to skip over the first part of the verse. The irony is that many people hang on to this scripture so tightly, when the desire of their heart seems to be overpowering them, but what the scripture actually says is that when you make the Lord your joy and desire him above all else, then He will give you the other desires of your heart.

- God taught me to rest in Him. Psalm 37 has so many wonderful verses that are very encouraging. Like verse 7: *"Be still in the presence of the Lord, and wait patiently for him to act. Don't worry about evil people who prosper or fret about their wicked schemes."* Many times we can get so restless when we are waiting for something. If you're like me and try to plan everything, then it can extremely frustrating when waiting messes up your plans! Furthermore, it can be disheartening when you see other women get pregnant around you, especially those who aren't married and don't even want a baby.

- God showed me the power of His grace. Sometimes it feels overwhelming to want something so badly and yet have to wait so long for it. Yet, everyday God gives us the strength to make it through another day. *"The temptations in your life are no different from what others experience. And God is faithful. He will not allow the temptation to be more than you can stand. When you are tempted, he will show you a way out so that you can endure"* (1 Corinthians 10:13).

Sometimes you can appear to have it all, but not be fulfilled in your heart. That was my story when my angel—Cassandra Scott—came into my life. I was in a place where I felt an emptiness that was hard to describe and hard to understand. I didn't feel good about myself. I felt unfulfilled where I was in my life. I began to cry out to God Who heard me and inclined His ear unto me. His answer was packaged in the person of Cassandra Scott and the opportunity of Mary Kay Cosmetics.

Cassandra relit my light. She spoke life into me and showed me that there truly was greatness inside of me. She took me under her wings and coached me from the beginning of my journey until this present moment.

We had a scheduled time to work together for her to mentor me and for me to grow in my business. She, via long distance calls coached me to earn my first free career car and become a Sales Director in Mary Kay within my first months of starting my business. Her business savvy—coupled with her strong communication skills—never ceases to me amaze me. I am a living witness that if you do what your Independent Sales Director teaches you - you can be successful. She has the ability to vividly paint a picture of success and achievement that totally motivates me.

This amazing woman of God has an uncanny ability to breathe belief into you and encourage you to breathe belief into others. I honor God and truly thank Him for the gift to the earth and to my life called Cassandra Scott.

Respectfully Submitted,
Lady Patrice Smith

4
The Process of Waiting

Process: A series of actions or steps taken to achieve an end. I remember my mom saying, "We are going to Weiner's to get you clothes for school", I was so excited! But then she said, "I will put them on layaway and pay on them, but you won't get them until just before school starts." That was a bittersweet moment for me. I was happy sad. I wanted the clothes as I tried them on. I wanted to take them home when we left the store. Going to the store in great expectation to try things on that I liked was awesome, but putting them on the counter parting with them was another story. Now all I had was dreams and hopes that my mother would be able to make that last layaway payment.

I bragged to my friends about what I had. However, since they could not see what I saw, they simply gave me that "yea right" look.

Nonetheless, I had the hidden promise in my heart. The process of waiting almost drove me crazy, but my mom had to make payments to purchase what was promised. When I look back over my life, it seems everything I wanted was one long waiting process. This was the beginning process of my life at a turning point.

I remember when my pastor, Rev. Samuel H. Smith, of Mt. Horeb Baptist Church called me into his office and said to me, "You will be married to a minister."

I had my doubts. I didn't know any ministers that I would want to marry and God knew I didn't want a preacher, anyway. I was still singing in the choir and going to the club immediately after church for ladies night. I didn't want to marry a preacher, that didn't fit with my plans. Oh, but my God better. He knew the plans that He had for me. Around March 1985 or 1986, I met Rev. Gary E. Scott. Friends, it was love at first sight. The process of my life had reached another turning point.

Gary and I got married, and, soon after, I began dreaming of having my husband's first child. If you are a woman who has spent your life imagining what it would be like to have a child, then you know how exciting it is when you finally decide that you are ready to take that leap. You are finally prepared to put yourself second, you are willing to make that child the number one priority in life, and you are ready to get pregnant.

Now that I was a pastor's wife, the next thing people asked was, *"Do you want any children? When will you start? Do you want boys or girls?"* I didn't care what the sex of my babies was, I just wanted to produce.

After almost a year of asking the same questions, people kind of slacked off and began giving me those "What is the problem looks"? I was so embarrassed. I just kept saying, we are trying; smiling and frowning at them at the same time. If you are a woman who has tried repeatedly, and have been unable to conceive, then you also know the veritable barrage of emotions that you encounter; grief, embarrassment, and uselessness. The enemy tormented me day and night about my inability to conceive.

After nearly three years of marriage, I was ready. I can hardly remember a time when I didn't want to have children with Gary. I cannot remember a time, when I didn't daydream about being a mother. I feel very strongly that we are all on this planet for a very specific reason and I have always thought that my reason was being a mother. Every woman I knew was like a fertility machine, conceiving *every* time they tried; imagine my surprise when after a year of trying I still wasn't pregnant. Frustration began to set in, *Why me?* I wondered.

It reminded me of those layaway payments at Weiner's for my school clothes, when my mom said that I had to wait. This, for me, was déjà vu. Instead of making payments on clothes, now we were paying to have a child. We were making payments, but couldn't get the child we both wanted so badly. How can so many people get pregnant the one time they have unprotected sex, and I'm doing everything suggested by doctors, old wives tales, myths, and the woman down the street who has eight kids, and still not conceive.

When you spend a year trying to conceive and are unable, it is often considered an early sign of infertility. You (and your partner) are then subjected to every test under the sun, most of which involve full or partial nudity in front of one or more people. Some things are too embarrassing to mention. Another year goes by, I start to feel guilty. My husband and I had always planned to have children. The doctors believed it was likely that something in *my* body was causing the problem.

I began to question my purpose as a woman. I can say with absolute certainty that my husband did not hold an ounce of contempt or blame for me, but that did not hold off the guilt and feelings of uselessness that I felt nonetheless. Feelings of guilt rear their ugly heads on a daily basis and at the worst times. With the guilt comes the worst feeling of all; begrudging the people around you the same happiness you want for yourself, because you want so desperately to have a child and cannot.

One of my friends called me and announced that she was pregnant. As I listened on the phone, I tried to fix my voice. I was simultaneously happy for her and extremely bitter about my inability to conceive. When I attended her baby shower, it was torturous experience. Because I not only I felt angry that things were going so good for her, but I also felt like a heinous person for having those selfish thoughts at all. I was angry at everyone, mostly myself.

The kicker in all of this is stress, which, if you let it, makes it even harder to conceive. After three years into the process (because that's exactly what it's become–a process) and realizing no results, I allowed stress to overwhelm me.

The key is acknowledging that you are angry, sad or depressed. Once you do, you validate the feelings and they are no longer so desperate. I urge every woman or couple out there to do the same. Talk to each other. Talk to someone else. Write a blog or join a support group. Whatever you do, know you that are not the only one, even if it feels that way.

Trying to conceive was very stressful and lead to feelings of anxiety and depression. I knew that one day I would conceive, but the waiting process is what I didn't like. As the months passed by without a positive pregnancy test, I sat and looked at that test and tried to change that negative to a positive in my mind. I had to find a support group.

My doctor recommended fertility experts, as a way of preventing the situation from getting too distressing, and there is evidence that doing so could actually improve your chances of conception. If your life revolves around a strict routine of basal body temperature monitoring and scheduled sex, consider taking a break because you will not get the promise, until due season. I read that fertility experts agree that charting or using ovulation prediction kits to time intercourse can make the whole process of trying to conceive even more stressful; and there is no evidence that these methods improve chances of conceiving naturally anyway. I made an effort to revive the love and fun that brought my husband and me together in the first place.

Because I was married to a pastor, we were often invited to certain gatherings and celebrations. This was painful for me. The birthday parties for young relatives and church members, Christenings for my friends' babies and the seemingly endless baby showers. Publically, I had to smile, of course, and pretend that I was happy for all of them, but I felt so empty and uncomfortable inside. Sometimes I would give myself permission to miss occasionally; especially when my emotions were all over the place. At the other end of the spectrum, having a good cry had a therapeutic effect, so boy did I cry; letting those feelings out made me feel better.

I want to reach out to those of you who haven't been able to produce, whether it is a child or something else that you don't have manifestation of. Infertility of any kind can be a lonely place—I know I've walked that road, too. I've had my times of sobbing in private after a friend, co-worker, or church member told me she's expecting. I would rant at God, "It's unfair that I can't have a child, when there are all sorts of people who don't even care about You, yet they have no problem at all!" And finally, those painful Mother's Day church services; as I watched all the beaming mothers stand up around me, it represented a club that I would never be a member of.

Pastor Cassandra Evett Scott and I have been friends since Pre-kindergarten. I remember it like yesterday: It was our first year in school; the teacher placed us at a small table as we each came in on the first day of school. "San" sat on the end at the table and I sat on the other side as we prepared to eat our snacks.

I asked her if she wanted one of my white donuts, and she smiled and said, "Yes." We have been friends ever since that day. We have shared so many firsts in life; we were in the same classes all throughout school. We were both born in Herman Hospital, in September, two days apart. I know our lives were destined by God. San and I are like sisters, we were cheerleaders, majorettes, band students, we both played the flute, and we were like two peas in a pod. You never saw one without the other.

I thank God for crossing our paths. It has been a wonderful life long journey for us, filled with many ups and downs, but we always had each other. We were both in church as young girls, very involved and we loved the Lord. We often studied the Bible together sitting at her mom's kitchen table, while Ms. Hilliard fixed greens, candied yams, and hot water cornbread. Ms. Hilliard told us, "Y'all better stop playing with God,"

Pastor C has helped me see what had become dormant in my ministry, and I thank God that she has lovingly reached out to me as the Big sister, and shared with me that we were Created 2 Produce. Her life is a true testimony; she is small in stature but mighty in spirit. Through partnering with her in ministry, I have experienced many firsts again, I have started a bible study, Transformation Ministries, and I have announced my call to the ministry. I love Pastor C and thank God that we are once again connected for life in ministry and Kingdom building. We break bread together in Pre-kindergarten and now through Christ Jesus, we break the Bread of Life together.

I love you San forever and always.

Veronica Harrison

5

Victory

Several years had passed since the miscarriage. Maybe my cup wasn't filled with what I wanted or the boundary lines hadn't fallen exactly as I planned, but they were assigned to me by the Creator of the universe, the most powerful God, the One who loves me and gave His life for me.

Maybe you're struggling with this issue today. No matter what you're going through, ask yourself: What's your Isaac? What is God asking you to surrender to Him today? What is it that you want more than you want God? I had to realize I was consumed with this desire more than my relationship with God. I repented, confessed, and put it under the blood of Jesus! And in almost no time – the nurses said to me from the charting of my BBT, *"Cassandra, You are pregnant!"*

I carried my first baby for 38 weeks. We named her Garelyn Evett Scott. She was so beautiful that the pain and the frustration were soon forgotten. God had answered my prayers! The doctor told me that if I ever wanted to have another child, I would have to go through fertility treatment again. I didn't think I wanted to go through that again.

Five years later, Gabrielle Chrishelle Scott was born, and two years after that, Gary Emerson Scott, II was born. I had a strong compassion to help others who went through this valley of the shadow of death. It was a feeling I can't describe. I wanted to help other women who desperately wanted children and weren't able to produce them. For me personally, not being able to conceive all those years was like a thorn in my flesh, and I wanted to help other women who were challenged with similar circumstances and pain to experience their victory.

Thus, I created a support group for women who were having difficulties conceiving. I remember teaching a women's Bible study class and speaking about conception. After the first lesson, seven women came to the front of the class. I laid hands on their wombs and prayed for them. Every three months, each of those women became pregnant, although their doctors had previously diagnosed them with various difficulties in conceiving.

At first, when the doctors announced that I was pregnant, I was stunned. I couldn't believe it. My doctor's office called, they instructed me to come in right away. "We want to do the pregnancy test because, even though the chart says, 'Yes,' we want to make sure. I was trembling like a leaf on a tree. I was so happy, but numb.

I rushed to the doctor's office, the nurses shouted for joy. They hugged and embraced me, and were overjoyed for me. I went into the room, undressed slowly and succumbed to all of the tests that were scheduled. Everything came back positive. I held my stomach and cried. I yelled, "Thank You Jesus!" I had finally conceived.

I wondered, *Am I carrying a girl or a boy?* Deep in my heart I wanted a girl.

My doctor gave me all of the Do's and Don'ts. She said, "The first three months, are the most critical time of your pregnancy, you are high risk. I remembered what happened before we had a miscarriage and those thoughts ran across my mind. I thought to myself, Would *this baby stick through the first trimester?* A bevy of emotions roared through me.

I bought a baby gift from the store and took it home. I handed to my husband. He looked at me in my eyes and said, *"Are You Pregnant?*

"Yes!" I exclaimed.

That was the happiest day of my life – God's hand opened my womb.

The pregnancy period marks remarkable changes in the woman's body - both mental and physical - some visible, others invisible. One must be equipped to tackle all these changes that accompany a pregnancy. Knowing and appreciating these changes can help one lead a better life during these nine months. I was changing from the inside out! Something inside said, *"Keep Quiet",* and then something else inside of me said, *"Tell the World".* I felt like an erupting volcano waiting to explode.

I thought back to the last time I was pregnant. I told everyone when I was only four weeks along and then I had a miscarriage. *Could this happen to me again?* I didn't know what to do, but believe for the best, so I told the world.

"V-I-C-T-O-R-Y" was a cheer we did when I was in school. Now was also appropriate. I was being transformed. I was changing from the inside out, I was created to produce, and knew that I would have the manifestation in nine months. What it would be like, who would it look like, so many questions, ran across my mind! This is huge, exciting news. I gave myself some time to revel my shared secret for a few days (or weeks). I picked a time to tell my parents and family and our church congregation. I broke the news to both sets of parents with similar timing and fanfare to avoid hurt feelings. As for my best friends, I said, "I'm pregnant! Let's party!"

Every week, I called my doctor and asked what was going on inside of me now. She always broke it down plain and simple. She gave me many books to read. I charted every day what I was feeling, how much I weighed each day (LOL), how I was changing and the baby! What I liked and disliked! It was amazing; no one could have done this but God!

What happens during each trimester?

Here is a snapshot of how my baby developed and how my body changed during each trimester of pregnancy. I loved to gage where I was in each trimester and what was actually happening.

First trimester (Weeks 0 to 13)

What happens to baby?

The sperm fertilizes the egg in the fallopian tube. The fertilized egg moves down the fallopian tube and attaches to the uterine wall.

All of the major organs and body structures - including the brain, heart, spinal cord and intestines - start to develop during the first half of this trimester.

Bones and muscles start to form. Muscles can contract and your baby can make a fist.

The baby weighs about one ounce and is about three inches long at the end of this stage.

What happens to you: Pregnancy-related hormone changes will start to affect your entire body. You may feel the effects of these changes before you even know you're pregnant. Some women experience the following conditions during the first trimester of pregnancy. But some women feel none at all:

Morning sickness

Weight gain

Exhaustion

Breast swelling and soreness

Cravings for certain foods or aversion to foods you usually like

Mood swings

Headaches

Need to urinate more frequently

Constipation

Second trimester (Weeks 14 to 27)

What happens to baby?

By the start of the second trimester, sex organs form. Your doctor may be able to tell if your baby is a boy or girl by now.

The placenta finishes developing.

The eyebrows, eyelashes and fingernails form. Your baby has his or her own unique fingerprint.

Your unborn baby can swallow, hear and suck his or her thumb.

The baby's body will be wrinkly and covered by a wax-like substance (vernix) and thin hair (lanugo). The baby's real hair will start to grow by the end of this trimester.

In girls, all of the eggs will develop in her ovaries. In boys, the testicles will drop down from the abdomen into the scrotum.

Your baby will start a regular sleep and wake cycle. He or she will be active during hours spent awake. You should be able to feel him or her move around and kick by the middle of the second trimester (at about 20 weeks).

The baby weighs a little over two pounds and is about 14 inches long.

What happens to you: By now, morning sickness and fatigue have often subsided. This is when you start "looking pregnant" as a result of your growing baby. You may experience the following discomforts as your body expands:

Body aches, especially in your back and abdomen

Stretch marks

Dry, itchy stomach

Tingly or numb hands

Slight swelling in your feet, fingers and face (if swelling comes on quickly, call your doctor because this could be a sign of preeclampsia)

A dark line running from your belly button to your pubic line, called the linea nigra.

Third trimester (Weeks 28 to 40)

What happens to baby?

Your baby grows the most during the third trimester.

The baby opens his or her eyes for the first time since the end of the first trimester. He or she can even notice changes in light.

The lanugo starts falling off at the start of this trimester. The skin will be less wrinkled.

The baby will likely descend down the uterus into the heads-down position to get ready for delivery.

Your baby's taste buds will form and he or she will be able to tell the difference between sweet and sour tastes. The baby may even hiccup.

All organs will be fully developed by the end of the third trimester.

At birth, your baby will be around 20 inches long and weigh between six and nine pounds. But healthy babies can come in all shapes and sizes.

What happens to you: You may be the most uncomfortable during the final stage of pregnancy. Because of your size, you may find it hard to get comfortable and sleep at night. In addition to what you felt during the second trimester, you may also experience:

Heartburn

Shortness of breath

Pre-milk called colostrum leaking from your nipples

Contractions that may signal real or false labor

I loved being pregnant. There were so many perks. Everyone lets you have your way; you are treated so kindly; everyone wants to wait on you, and lastly, one of the best perks of pregnancy is being able to blame things on pregnancy. I wanted to eat everything, and some things I didn't want to eat. If you don't feel like going to your weird cousin's costume party, you can say you're just too tired. Do you want another donut? Go for it. Amazing!

Congratulations, kudos, and woo hoo! You're pregnant! In those rare moments when you're not dancing on air or completely freaking out, you may be wondering what you need to do next. You begin to develop more wisdom; you learn how to become a leader – a parent – and a developer of the precious soils that has been entrusted to you.

My husband, Edward and I were told by a fertility specialist that we would not be able to have children because he had no sperm. It was devastating news and I just did not want to accept it. I later went to my OB/GYN for my annual exam and shared with her the news of my husband's infertility. She gave me a name of a fertility specialist for men, but cautioned me that it was extremely expensive. In addition, she told me to just get a sperm donor. I left her office in shock, and couldn't believe what she had said.

I went through the In-Vitro process and had support from members of the Fruitful Womb Ministry and Pastor C. She had prayed, laid hands on, and provided spiritual guidance to me. Well, needless to say, I did conceive! When I called Pastor C to tell her she was elated. She was so happy for me and she began to praise God. She asked me about the details, and I shared with her that the doctor had transferred two embryos and her response was, "Double for your trouble!" Later, I discovered that I was only having one child....a girl. I reminded Pastor C that it was at the Fruitful Womb Ministry that her teenage daughter had prophesied that I was going to have a girl! I was so excited and grateful that she listened to the Holy Spirit and allowed her daughter to flow in the anointing on that day.

When my daughter, Sarah, was born on July 25, Pastor C made it to the hospital. I was overjoyed and felt so special that she took time out to celebrate with me. Well, a few years passed and Pastor C was no longer at Trinity. However, I would communicate with her through text messages. Even though Pastor C ministered and counseled me through this ministry, it was what she did afterwards that has extremely impacted me. I now have twin girls ("double for my trouble"), Victoria and Elizabeth who are 2 and Sarah is now 6. Pastor C is truly a remarkable woman in ministry and I pray that God continues to bless her and use her to advance His Kingdom!

Tyra Stemley

6

Ready, Aim, Fire

Proverbs 22:6 - New International Version (NIV) ⁶ Start children off on the way they should go, and even when they are old they will not turn from it.

I didn't realize that my mom was pointing us as arrows in the right direction. My mom said "Open your mouth and sing when I hit the key on the piano." As scared as I was, I opened my mouth and before I knew it, I was singing. She placed us on Coke carts so people could see us. I was somewhere between four- or five-years-old. We had many engagements, even when we didn't want them, they still became available.

We had no choice to say what we would, or wouldn't do. We knew nothing of child protective services (CPS). Naomi was CPS in my view. She said, "If you don't open your mouth when it's time, I'm gonna get off the piano and whip your butt." I thought to myself, *this lady is crazy*, but I wasn't gonna take the chance and be whipped in front of the entire congregation.

I would almost hate when people came over, she would say, "Ken, San, Rocky, come in here and sing for such and such."

We could be in a deep sleep, when she was ready; we had better be ready too. She would say to everyone, so proudly, "My kids can sing." I would sink inside my soul, hoping she would just shut up; nobody wants to hear me and my brothers sing. They came over to visit you, and now we are in concert. I didn't want to do another performance for anyone, I was shy, didn't know who I was; and didn't seem to fit in with a lot of children.

Not only natural parents, but spiritual parents will point you in the right direction. Many spiritual fathers and mothers have been responsible for gearing people to their destiny. You must pray and ask God to show you who your spiritual parents are. Many children's destiny and gifts have been aborted, because some parents were not aware who they were naturally and/or spiritually. They may have been too religious to hear the order of God, or they were too jealous, self centered, and selfish to mentor, coach and train others. 1 Samuel 16:7-13 - (NIV) [7] But the LORD said to Samuel, "Do not consider his appearance or his height, for I have rejected him. The LORD does not look at the things people look at. People look at the outward appearance, but the LORD looks at the heart." [8] Then Jesse called Abinadab and had him pass in front of Samuel. But Samuel said, "The LORD has not chosen this one either." [9] Jesse then had Shammah pass by, but Samuel said, "Nor has the LORD chosen this one." [10] Jesse had seven of his sons pass before Samuel, but Samuel said to him, "The LORD has not chosen these." [11] So he asked Jesse, "Are these all the sons you have?" "There is still the youngest," Jesse answered. "He is tending the sheep." Samuel said, "Send for him; we will not sit down until he arrives." [12] So he sent for him and had him brought in. He was glowing with health and had a fine appearance and handsome features. Then the LORD said, "Rise and anoint him; this is the one." 13 So Samuel took the horn of oil and anointed him in the presence of his brothers, and from that day on the Spirit of the LORD came powerfully upon David. Samuel then went to Ramah.

If your natural parents are not spiritual enough to see the call of God on your life, God will send a Samuel anointing, to be sensitive enough in the spirit to send for you; one that spends much time in prayer to anoint you and to point you in the right direction. It will be public, so all your relatives and friends can see. Those who thought you were not qualified will now have to watch you get elevated! Those that are last – shall be first! Jeremiah 29:11 - (NIV) 11 For I know the plans I have for you," declares the LORD, "plans to prosper you and not to harm you, plans to give you hope and a future. There will be people put in our life, to point you in the right direction. You are Created 2 Produce, everything you need inside of you has already been made available; the connection just needs to be made! Psalms 127:4, *"Like arrows in the hand of a warrior, so are children of one's youth."* Every child needs a virtuous bow, like Lois and Eunice who taught their offspring from childhood the Holy Scriptures (II Timothy 3:15; 1:5); and like the woman described in Proverbs 31:10-31. Like arrows, children need two distinct and different external aids -- an archer (father) and bow (mother). Without an archer, an arrow never takes flight. Without a bow, an arrow can be nothing more than a puny spear. By divine design, every child has a father (its archer) and a mother (its bow). The accuracy and force that an arrow has is largely dependent upon the aim and strength of the archer, and the integrity and caliber of the bow. My parents were surely the archer and bow!

Like arrows, children must be aimed and released. Like arrows, children are a one shot deal. Like arrows, children have great potential for good and evil. Few things in life are more devastating and depressing than the regrets of careless, foolish, shortsighted parents. Consider what heartache God says awaits them: "*He who begets a scoffer does so to his sorrow, and the father of a fool has no joy*" (Proverbs 17:21). Our world has been blessed with archers and bows in the bible, which were responsible for pointing their child or individuals into destiny: Naomi and Ruth, Elizabeth and Mary, Mordecai and Esther, Zacaraus and Elizabeth (John), Joseph and Mary (Jesus), and Amram and Jocebed (Moses). There are turning point moments that are destined in each of our lives. I thought, because of my natural rearing, that I didn't have a chance until the word became alive in me. Raised in a single family home on welfare, without transportation, statistics put me in a category of less likely to succeed. My twelfth grade teacher looked me in the eyes and told me, "I would never make it in the front of the whole class", I was crushed! I could never explain how embarrassed I was, I could hardly lift up my head. I thought what had I done to deserve such cruel words! Somebody lied when they said, "Sticks and stones can break my bones; but words will never hurt me". People will be sent into your life to shatter your dreams and visions, but lift your head up and stand on the word of God. This is an indication you are on the right road, don't give up! Stand up and open your mouth and profess the living Word of the Lord! I just knew that I wasn't like everyone else and didn't want to do what everyone else did. Jesus was calling me, but I didn't really know it! Spiritual Mentors, Teachers, Pastors, etc., were sent into my life at the right time to experience different turning points; like Bishop Ira and Pastor Bridget Hilliard, Pastor S. H. Smith, Doris Scott, Deacon Frank and Alyce Kinney, Apostle Corletta Vaughn, Pastor Connie Brooks, Bishop David and Pastor Claudette Copeland and countless others to point me in the right direction. Rest assured God knows who your parents should be spiritually and naturally to get you to the place you were Created 2 Produce.

Just as God wants to point you and I in the right direction, the adversary will send people to get us off course. I remember people who were sent to get me off course! They came in all shapes, forms and sizes. Just as Potipher's wife came to Joseph, to cause him to actually abort the plan of God; she was sent to cause him to be pointed in the opposite direction. The bible explains in Genesis 39:7…"And after a while his master's wife took notice of Joseph and said, "Come to bed with me!" Has anyone ever asked you that question? Guess what? It was an assignment to point you in the wrong direction, to hinder the plan of God for your life. There is nothing new under the sun and someone is taking

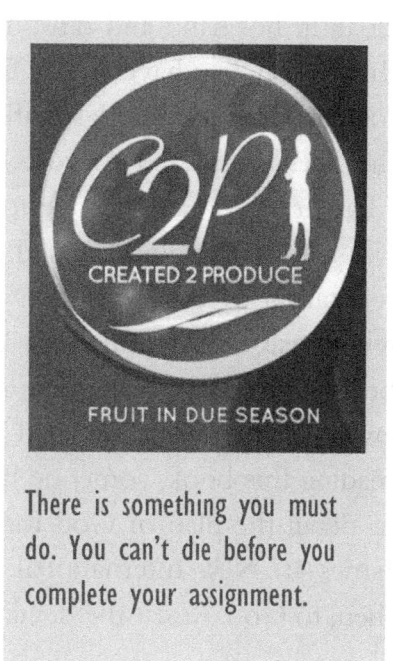

There is something you must do. You can't die before you complete your assignment.

notice of you! 1 Corinthians 10:11 -New International Version (NIV) 11 These things happened to them as examples and were written down as warnings for us, on whom the culmination of the ages has come. She already had her eye on Joseph and "day after day" it was the same response, "No". Genesis 39:10 says, "And though she spoke to Joseph day after day, he refused to go to bed with her or even be with her." The last time Potiphar's wife insisted, she managed to get a piece of his coat, which she kept as evidence against Joseph. The bible says... "She caught him by his cloak and said, "Come to bed with me!" but he left the cloak in her hand and ran out of the house (Genesis 39:12). In this season, you have to flee for your life, there are others waiting for you to get to the destination marked by God for you, and all the lives connected to you. Potiphar's wife was the Proverbs Chapter 7 woman, the one to be real careful with. This woman was full of lust, and she didn't care what happened to Joseph's reputation or destiny. I have seen countless men and women with great callings on their life get sidetracked in this area. I believe the bible has pointed this story out to all of us for awareness as we are headed in the right direction. As you are reading this book, someone has been assigned to you, to get you to derail the plan of God for your destiny and countless others. James 4:7 New International Version (NIV) 7 Submit yourselves, then, to God. Resist the devil, and he will flee from you.

There is something that you must do. You can't die before you complete your assignment. You must resist the enemy. This will be your turning point. Everything you need has already been provided, this is your turning point you are Created 2 Produce. Someone said, the riches place in the world is the cemetery many dreams, lawyers, doctors, presidents, scientist, pastors, writers, millionaires, etc., have died with their dreams inside of them with hidden talents in darkness. I love the story of David, taking care of the sheep, doing what he did best, fighting lions and bears without an audience; just making it happen in the due season. Samuel, the prophet shows up, and in one day he is elevated and pointed like an arrow in the right direction– no one recognized him before – but God knew he was Created 2 Produce. He will send the right people in your life that will recognize the call of God on your life, and create the atmosphere for you to walk into your destiny. All you need is that one person assigned by God to show up and point you in the right direction and the rest will be history. Each of us are Created 2 Produce, once we are born and enter into this world, there is a certain assignment that God has for you to complete. We each have been placed in a garden by God and he wants us to be fruitful and multiply. This scripture is the one scripture that has totally set me free – all of my past self esteem issues died – once I trained myself to meditate on this scripture: I am created in the very image of God.

This is liberating to my soul, body and spirit. I don't just read over this scripture, I have meditated it. "The fact that man is the image of God means that man is like God in some of the following ways: intellectual ability, moral purity, spiritual nature, dominion over the earth, creativity, ability to make ethical choices, and immortality." Genesis 1:26-28 - New International Version (NIV) 26 Then God said, "Let us make mankind in our image, in our likeness, so that they may rule over the fish in the sea and the birds in the sky, over the livestock and all the wild animals, [a] and over all the creatures that move along the ground." ²⁷ So God created mankind in his own image, in the image of God he created them; male and female he created them. ²⁸ God blessed them and said to them, "Be fruitful and increase in number; fill the earth and subdue it. Rule over the fish in the sea and the birds in the sky and over every living creature that moves on the ground. I realized that God breathed into me. Everything I went through was for the development of my character and destiny. I had to die so that Christ could live. I fell in love with God for real. I wasn't pretending church anymore; I wasn't into religion, but relationship.

Dr. Cassandra Scott and I met at a Mary Kay Business meeting in 2003. Later, she asked me to become her parents' primary care physician. It was an honor to care for their health care needs. Our sisterhood bond flourished to this day and I'm committed to supporting her Kingdom Vision.

In July 2010, Dr. Scott invited me to encourage the callers on the CSM 6am prayer call. They were in their 2nd shift of 40 days of praying. It transformed our lives! Dr. Scott ministry has encouraged me to start my own weekly leadership call, "Take God as your Business Partner". Also, a monthly student leadership call named, "Operation Soar". Where I teach students to stay focused on their God given purpose.

CSM is now an International Prayer call transforming lives for the Glory of God! While growing Butterfly Wellness, non-profit for women who need mammograms, the 6am call led me to accept the position Medical Director of a wellness center that also serves those suffering with HIV/AIDs. This is a new territory that God led me to serve his people. Now, I'm planning international missionary trips to share the message of Jesus Christ and to open HIV clinics in 3rd World Countries.

The prayer line under Dr. Scott's leadership has taught us to teach people how to live a life of Prayer and Obedience! We are on a rescue mission to seek and save lives! It was all God's plan that we would meet at a business meeting, and I would become their family physician, then go on divine assignments with Dr. Scott to deliver God's message!

I'm Created 2 Produce,
Love
Dr. Sabrina Echols

7
Girl Interrupted

Pregnancy. There are approximately 6 million pregnancies each year throughout the United States. Of which, a little more than 4 million result in live births.

Abortion. The loss of an embryo or fetus either spontaneously (miscarriage) or induced (when a pregnancy is terminated on purpose) before 20 weeks. After 20 weeks, the spontaneous loss of a fetus is called a stillbirth.

Pregnancy Loss. Nearly 2 million women experience a loss during pregnancy by still birth, ectopic pregnancy or miscarriage; I believe this happens spiritually as well. What have you birthed that was stillborn, an ectopic pregnancy, or miscarriage or even a lost? It almost killed you; you got rid of it, but you are still here with the memory of being pregnant in the spirit, but never holding your dream. You had to bury what you know God intended for your life.

Pregnancy Complications. Almost a million other women in the United States experience one or more pregnancy complications, e.g., infertility, low birth weight or birth defect which appears to impact most women between the ages of 30 and 39 years. How many of us have had complications, you knew that you were suppose to do something for God, but you were infertile, had low birth weight ministries and ministries that had birth defects? You had complications like layoffs, divorce, illness, trouble with children, etc.

1 Corinthians 15:46: NIV ⁴⁶ The spiritual did not come first, but the natural, and after that the spiritual. I believe this has happened to many of us. We have experienced spiritual pregnancy loss, complications, attempts to abort the plan of God and kill us once we have birthed. People have been sent to kill what you did deliver because of the anointing on our lives.

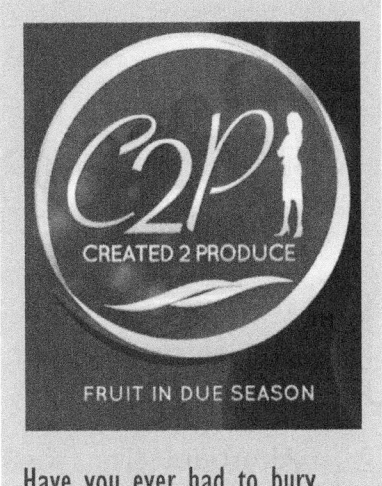

Have you ever had to bury what you know God intended for your life?

Exodus 1: NIV ¹⁵ The king of Egypt said to the Hebrew midwives, whose names were Shiphrah and Puah, ¹⁶ "When you are helping the Hebrew women during childbirth on the delivery stool, if you see that the baby is a boy, kill him; but if it is a girl, let her live." ¹⁷ The midwives, however, feared God and did not do what the king of Egypt had told them to do; they let the boys live. Many men and women who have a call on their lives, attempted to produce, but there is a King of this world commanding your ministry, family, business, etc., be killed as soon as you deliver it. Don't give up and don't quit, your help is on the way; this is your turning point! There will be midwives in the spirit, who will be sent to help you push out that hidden treasure inside of you. God will send people who are assigned to you, to resuscitate you, so you can be all that God has designed.

When you are Created 2 Produce, get ready to wait. There's a waiting room where our dreams go between inception and realization. God allows this period of waiting to see if we will stoke the fire of our dream, or if we'll let the spark die out.

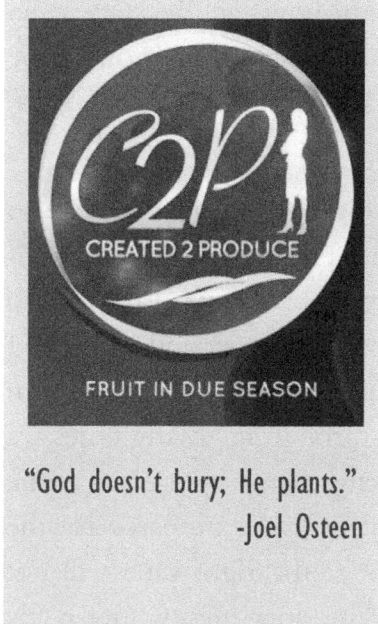

"God doesn't bury; He plants."
-Joel Osteen

I can't count the number of people over the years, who have told me in a fit of emotion that they will become a missionary, a pastor, they will start a ministry for homeless people, young people, old people, single people, poor people, or start a business. They're completely enthusiastic about the idea for about three days, and then they forget about it.

I couldn't stop thinking about holding my first child. At first, I thought it was just about wanting a child, but now I see it was part of my destiny. Not being able to conceive when I wanted to was preparing me for the people I was called to be a witness to. I wasn't there in my relationship with God then that made no sense to me then. When God gives you a dream, He will give that dream the opportunity to incubate in your heart for a while. Oh how it incubated. I thought for a minute; *forget it*, because it was taking too long. Have you ever wanted something so bad and it seemed like everyone else was getting what you wanted. Even when it seemed that you had to bury it because the dream was dead. A friend of mine recently shared with me this Joel Osteen quote, "Remember, God doesn't bury; He plants." God will give it time to grow. You can expect to spend some time waiting.

When you are Created 2 Produce, get ready for the open door. If God has given you a dream, you can be sure—even though it may seem like things are on hold right now—you can be sure that God will provide an open door when the time is right. The question is: Will you be ready?

Start asking yourself these questions: What do I need to do in order to get this thing started? What information should I gather? What facts do I need to know? Which skills do I need to learn? Who are the people who can help me most and who will I be working with? Start asking these questions now, so that when the door is open, you're ready to go through it. Many times we attribute success to being lucky, or being in the right place at the right time. Luck will not help you unless you're prepared for the opportunity. Being in the right place at the right time will not help you, unless you're prepared for the opportunity. Get ready for the open door. It won't be long before it swings wide; make sure you're in a position to go through not just a single door but a double door!

"Production interruptions always require a call to leadership."

-Merle Ray

When you are Created 2 Produce, get ready to spend time in prayer. If God has given you a dream to lead in a certain area, to accomplish a certain task, begin praying about it now. Ask God to make you clean, to give you pure motives, to give you wisdom to make the right decisions, to give you courage to face opposition, to give you humility, integrity and patience and discernment, to keep your ego in check, to provide everything you need, and to guide you with his hand day after day after day. Make everything a matter of prayer. If you're already in a position of leadership, and you're not praying like you ought to be praying, start today. Start this moment. Start with a bullet prayer: "God, help me get my prayer life where it should be." And get in the habit of praying; it's an essential part of preparation. When my dreams and hopes crashed, like never before, I developed a prayer life of fasting and prayer. Because of prayer it has taken me places I never would have been able to go.

When you are Created 2 Produce, get ready for some late and lonely nights. There will come a time when you're ready to talk about your dream, but during the preparation process, it's best to keep it to yourself. During the preparation process, you can expect to spend some late nights all alone—thinking, planning, gathering information, evaluating, praying, thinking some more, developing a strategy, praying some more, until the time you are ready to move forward. The fact is that no one will know about the late nights. No one will know about the extra hours. No one needs to know. Leaders understand that we're the ones to arrive early and leave late. Leaders make preparation that no one sees. Leaders carry a burden that no one else feels. Leaders spend more time with a project than the spectators—or even the average participants—will ever realize.

Do you ever watch the Olympics? According to USA Today, the average Olympian trains four hours a day, 310 days a year, for six years, before making it to the Olympics. In training, swimmers average 10 miles a day in laps; marathon runners average 160 miles a week. They pay the price for their success; every successful leader must do the same. Preparation for leadership requires long days and late nights. These times when no one is cheering you on; the only thing that is driving you is the will to accomplish something great for the glory of God.

When you are Created 2 Produce, get ready for some opposition. Nehemiah didn't argue with his critics. So why do you? He didn't present them with his business plan or assure them the king was on his side, or try to convince them that his strategy would work. He just said, "This is God's project and he will give us success. This doesn't involve you at all ... so keep your nose out of it." Nehemiah shows us how to do it: with as few words as possible. I have never closed my mouth as much in the last 3-4 years. The important thing is to keep focused on what God is calling you to do, not what your opponents are saying.

Process can be difficult. It can be long and it can be lonely. But when you prepare God can use you. He *will* use you. He's given you a dream of making a difference -- at work, at home, in your community, in the ministry, etc. As you prepare your heart and life, he will take you to the place he has called you to be.

My attitude had to change. I was very bitter, jealous and angry with myself, God and others that I would see. I was standing in my own way, I was blocking my blessings – make sure it's not you standing in the way vs. a Sanballat or Tobiah, who opposed Nehemiah. The opposition can also come from you.

Active labor: Part of the first stage of labor when the cervix dilates from three to seven centimeters. Active labor lasts an average of two to four hours. The contractions during active labor are strong, long (40 to 60 seconds each), and frequent (three to four minutes apart). My faith had to shift; God would do it in His timing. My mind needed to be renewed. Renewing your mind is not just a suggestion, it actually brings your world into focus, (Romans 12:1-2) "I beseech you therefore, brethren, by the mercies of God, that you present your bodies a living sacrifice, holy, acceptable to God, which is your reasonable service. And be not conformed to this world, but be you transformed by the renewing of your mind, that you may prove what is that good, and acceptable and perfect, will of God." Start thinking as the Bible tells you, you are, (Ephesians 1:3) "blessed be the God and Father of our Lord Jesus Christ, who has blessed us with all spiritual blessings in heavenly places in Christ," it said, "we are blessed with all spiritual blessings."

Wrap your mind around that, and look at the fact that there is no sickness, poverty or tears in heaven. Jesus said "take no thought"(Matthew 6:31), saying when you speak you activate what you believe (Mark 11:23-24). "Whosoever shall say to this mountain, be you removed, and be you cast into the sea, and shall not doubt in his heart, but shall believe that those things which he says shall come to pass, he shall have whatsoever he says. Therefore I say to you, what things so ever you desire, when you pray, believe that you receive them, and you shall have them."Romans 4:17 "even God, who makes alive the dead, and calls those things which be not as though they were." We are told to be "imitators of God as dear children" (Ephesians 5:1). One of the things that limits us and keeps us defeated is the opinion we have of ourselves. Over time, we begin to accept that we can't change. We also accept other people's stigmas of us. These things begin to shape our view of ourselves and what we're capable of. My opinion was not what it should have been, I was very unsure of myself, and had very low self esteem! I thought, oh well – So you don't want to bless me God with a child – forget it – I don't want it – I was getting angry at God because it seemed to not work out in the right time for me. I thought I will just get over it.

Often we end up living up to the very opinions and expectations that others have had of us. We feel, *"I'll always be average." "I'll always be overweight." I'll never have a baby" "I'm capable of only making 'x' amount of money."* We're limited by our self-imposed expectations of ourselves. I needed to break out of the limitations and boundaries I had put on myself. The enemy was saying to me, "You will never conceive."

I realized:

I was a work of art—a work in progress. God is the potter and we are the clay (Jeremiah 18:1-6). I had to trust the Artist to make a masterpiece. I had to be flexible and adaptable. See myself as a good work in progress.

I had to stop withholding judgment of myself (or others). Philippians 1:6 says, "He who began a good work in you will complete it until the day of Jesus Christ." Don't prejudge what your capacity is or what your potential is, He's only just begun!

God doesn't throw you out. He never gives up on you. Jeremiah 18:4 says, "The clay was marred, so He made it again." He didn't discard it. He made it again. Whew! Thank God. Thank you He was making me all over. I was in the process and needed to embrace it. I was so use to people throwing me away when they were done!

I was changing and being transformed. I was Created 2 Produce and didn't even know it. Whatever flaws I have, they are not the final sentence. I was being conformed to the image of Jesus! (Romans 8:29)

Finally, embrace the grace. Paul said in 1 Corinthians 15:10, "I am what I am by the grace of God." It's God's grace in you that is making you what you are. You are not a composite of your parents' mistakes, your mistakes, and others' opinions of you. You're awesome.

In 2000, we moved from New Orleans to Houston and became members of Trinity Fellowship Church in 2001. There, we met Pastor Cassandra Scott, who we learned prayed for women who wanted to conceive. I joined the "Fruitful Womb Ministry." It was a great fellowship of women desiring to conceive. We had prayer partners and monthly fellowships. It was a wonderful time of encouragement. We laughed, cried and prayed together. There was nothing like talking to another woman who understood the journey of infertility. Pastor C was always available to talk us through a difficult time, to give a word of encouragement, help calm fears and most definitely to pray. She wanted us to birth what God had inside of us just as much as we did.

On our journey, because I knew the doctor recommended in-Vitro fertilization and we were well aware of how expensive it is, I told the Lord that He'd either do this naturally or give us the money to conceive. Well, he gave us the money for in-Vitro fertilization. We had success our first round! I was pregnant with twins. We had a few extremely frightening times during my pregnancy. I miscarried one of the twins very early and continued to bleed throughout the first trimester. At the first ultrasound, we discovered that my son had polycystic kidneys and one was not functioning. I even had a kidney specialist speak "fetal demise" over my son. At the end of the pregnancy, the blood stopped flowing through the umbilical cord. However, through all of the challenges, God was faithful and allowed us to be the proud parents of a wonderful son, Troy Jr. I remember Pastor C visiting me at the hospital. She was faithful and committed to walking this journey with us- and for that, I'm forever grateful.

We may never understand why we have to endure some of the things that God allows. But always remember that He has a plan. He has servants set up in the earth to help us along our journey. I believe that Pastor C's prayers extended beyond my son and included my daughter and that process as well. I would have never thought that I would have to have in-Vitro to conceive and then adopt to add to my family. Just because things do not happen in the manner we desire, many times we tend to reject them. I would encourage you to not reject how God wants to produce in you. I can testify that my acceptance of His plan and will for my life has tremendously added to my life and my family's life.

Antonio Moore

8
Identity Crisis

Mt. Zion MBC: I am a pastor's wife. I was just trying to fit in. I didn't know where I belonged. It was so scary. Being in this type of position, people try to make you fit their blue print for you – most times without even considering Gods original plan. If you are not careful, you will be dressed in someone else's armor, and that makes your movement almost confined. Guess what, I didn't fit in at all. I was absolutely comfortable with being under the umbrella of my former husband. I thought He fit the description and I'll just walk along in his shadow. Those were my thoughts because I surely didn't want to do anything else. I didn't even know if I could be a first lady. Who would train and coach me for this position? I was an introvert. I didn't know how to mix and mingle with people, and I had only two friends throughout elementary to high school. Who were all of these people who all of a sudden just showed up in our lives as our new family? I was fine when it was just us.

My former husband would say, "We are going to this function or that function," and I froze up inside. I thought, *What will I wear? How was my hair? Did my outfit look ok? Would they accept me as they accepted him?* I was so worried about the outward appearance. But God had a plan now to start bringing my true purpose to the forefront. I was getting closer to my turning point. When we would get in the company of people, I thought, "Lord please don't let him leave me". If he would just hold my hand, I felt I could make it. He seemed to be able to talk to people we didn't even know. I thought to myself, *How do you do that?*

I was devastated. I couldn't think of one word to say to people I didn't know. I didn't realize that these were turning point moments for me for development for where God was taking me. They asked me to teach children's Sunday school; I almost fainted. I wanted to change my membership. I couldn't eat for days. I thought, *if they would just leave me alone.* Our first church was connected to our parsonage, I would immediately go home after church and look out the window at all of the people laughing and talking to each other. I just didn't know how to do that. Jesus! I needed so much training. I didn't want to do any of that.

The one thing I did know how to do was what my mom trained me to do – sing. So I thought it was safe to stay in that lane in the choir. But my circle was enlarging and increasing. I was very uncomfortable. Later I realized, when you are uncomfortable it's because your season for producing is changing. I was pregnant spiritually and didn't even know it. You must know that God wants you to move to the next level in him. What worked at one season in your life was good; it was needed, but now God is getting you on his agenda to complete your assignment. I remember falling on my knees in the parsonage one Sunday after church, and asking God to anoint me for his service. I remember hearing people like Bettye Ransom Nelson and Kathy Taylor, every time they stood, it seemed the earth shook. My eyes would well up in tears, it pierced my soul. The power was undeniable.

I said God, "Would you give me what you gave them?" I reached out to Bettye Ransom Nelson and she actually started mentoring me and deposited belief and confidence that I originally didn't have as a first lady. On the journey, God will allow certain people to deposit into you. It reminded me of Elizabeth and Mary, when Mary realized she was pregnant, she went to spend a certain amount of time with her cousin; who was further along pregnant than she was. When they came into the presence of one another; what Elizabeth was pregnant with, leaped at Mary's arrival.

You need to connect with people who make your baby leap. There are certain people I get around and nothing happens. Then there are those who are further along than you, and have proof of their calling, which makes you want to literally jump out of the boat without any thought or security. I closed my eyes, and believed that He deposited inside of me, before the foundation of the earth. I said to myself, God said that he has no respect of persons, so If I didn't get the anointing to do His service, I told God I didn't or wouldn't do his work. I must have the oil and the anointing to make a difference. I wanted proof of my calling, I wanted signs and wonders. How many of you know that you are a *sign* and a *wonder*? People are wondering how you made it over after all you had to go through. You are also a sign that will lead people in the right direction.

Trinity Fellowship Houston Church: The ministry was spreading across the city and states by leaps and bounds. During those twenty-one years I learned so much. The journey was so God. I met so many people. Our life was totally blessed from the Lord. We started with nothing in the natural but big faith in God and had dreams of succeeding in life. So many people lives were blessed, healed, delivered and set free. Families, finances and faith were increasing by leaps and bounds in the lives of people. We went from looking outside many nights at the stars dreaming of what it would be like to walking in the will of God. Nobody knew us. Would anyone believe us and give us a chance?

We both grew up in the traditional Baptist church. We had a dream. It was not in the box we had been confined in. We were expecting and God blessed us to actually holding four churches in our hands. I believe God wanted us to be fruitful, multiply and take dominion at every season. We were blessed with Mt. Zion, Trinity Fellowship North, Trinity Fellowship South and Trinity Fellowship Florida, not to mention the community outreach and services, workshops, conferences, etc. We held the manifestation of what God had planned all along; everything working together for our good. Souls were being saved, baptisms were beyond number, ministries were being birthed and so much more. God said if we took care of His big business, He would take care of our little business. He absolutely did just what He said.

Matthew 6:33 says, "But seek ye first the kingdom of God, and his righteousness; and all these things shall be added unto you". It was added. We went from no car, home, money, to having exceedingly and abundantly above what we could ask or believe. It was without any effort. During this time in my life is where I started walking closer to producing all that God had dreamed for me. I thank God this day for the journey. I stand amazed.

You are expecting: This is where my life totally shifted. I was expecting spiritually. I was given the awesome opportunity to teach the women's ministry at Trinity weekly. Wow, I could not only sing as most first ladies, but now I was beginning to walk in the five fold ministry gifts. I was also a teacher.

Remember the first lady that was scared to talk to people? Now I was teaching many women on a monthly basis. It just seemed to flow. The anointing always showed up. People were testifying of the awesome blessings that was manifesting in their lives. I'll never forget I taught on "Being Pregnant Naturally and Spiritually." After teaching this lesson, the Holy Spirit led me to ask if there was anyone who was trying to conceive, or if and the doctor had diagnosed that you could not produce; about seven ladies ran to the front of the church.

As they were coming forth, I heard God say to me, "Each of them that believe will conceive." It was absolutely amazing. I laid my right hand on each of their belly, and God said for me to say out loud, "every three months each of them would conceive", if they only believed. The devil immediately started saying to me, don't you dare say that, it can't happen. The doctor has already told them that they can't produce.

I dared to do what God told me. Scared, I opened up my mouth and said, "You shall have a fruitful womb within 3 months each of you shall conceive". It happened just like I had said.

That was the beginning of God showing me that He would use me to pray for people all over the world to produce what was diagnosed by man – barren. I didn't even know I was expecting at this point spiritually, I was pregnant as well; spiritually God was shifting me into destiny. I went from now teaching weekly to also having a weekly prayer meeting from house to house in the city. It was absolutely breathtaking what God did to all of the women who would dare to come I was expecting and manifesting a teaching ministry and prayer ministry now. Whether you know it or not, you are expecting right now or have manifested what God put inside of you. It is sometimes a single pregnancy, twin pregnancy, etc. But you better believe you are pregnant. You are expecting.

Trinity Fellowship Orlando Florida Church: I was able to fly once a month and minister the word of God in Orlando, Florida. God was increasing and enlarging my capacity and territory. As I look back at all the opportunities that were given to me by my former husband; and other ministries that invited me to minister, I was literally on training ground for where I am now. Trinity Florida was a beautiful group of people that absolutely loved the word of God. God will put people in your life to help you get to your destination. You can accept full hearted or come kicking and screaming like I did, but you will eventually be caught in the belly of the whale and God will deal with you until you are ready to surrender to his divine plan.

Miscarriage: The spontaneous and involuntary loss of a pregnancy before 20 weeks, estimated to occur in 15 to 20 percent of all pregnancies. Most miscarriages occur in the first 12 weeks of pregnancy, and many occur before a woman even knows she's pregnant. The slogan: "*The family that prays together, stays together*" is well known.

Gary and I experienced a miscarriage early in our marriage. To know that you are pregnant, feel the baby moving, have all the symptoms, and one day wake up and it is all gone, is devastating. This is how I felt after our divorce. Termination is another word for abortion. After being married for twenty-one years, I never dreamed of being divorced. It was like a miscarriage. It was like a death. I had to go through counseling, I sought help and I had to have intercessors around to stand in the gap for me.

When you experience a miscarriage you have to heal, you have to stay off your feet. The enemy hit our home like a ton of bricks. Thank God for people that He put in my life for that time and season: Pastor Connie Brooks, Bishop Ira and Pastor Bridget Hilliard, Bishop David and Pastor Claudette Copeland, Apostle Corletta Vaughn, and Pastor Liddie Owens. It was one of the most devastating times of my life. In a divorce, no one wins. No wonder in the Bible, God says "I hate divorce."

I believe it is because He knows how deep it flows. Everyone was hurt. I was hurt, my former husband was hurt, our kids, both of our families, and not to mention our church family and friends. It was like an earthquake, I went into deep depression. I didn't want to go to church, preach, teach, sing, pray or even see anyone. I was totally embarrassed. I was excited and sad when I would see people that we had prayed for, married them at the altar, and their marriages where still standing. I thought in my mind, "how is it that we could pray for others and not maintain ourselves?" As Johnny Enlow refers to in his book, The Seven Mountain Mantle, I believe God wants me to take the family mountain in prayer and provide services and support for people who have experienced divorce or considering divorce. I would love to have services for people who are considering divorce, who do not have the money to divorce; we would provide free services for them to come to my office. I would offer to pay for the divorce, under one condition, you must agree to complete our counseling services. The aim would be in hopes of reconciliation, if at all possible. We do know some relationships are beyond repair, if both parties are not willing to be on one accord.

God hates divorce because of what it does to the families involved; the devastation and suffering that result are highly displeasing to him. But in all of this He is still able to make all grace abound and bring what seems dead to life. Remember Lazarus was dead and stinking, but God raised him up for those who did not believe – God can still give you a life after divorce. In particular, God *hates* the suffering of the children involved in divorces. God *hates* it when a home is broken and a family shattered. God *hates* it when children are deprived of father or mother by divorce. God loathes the heartbreak of the children, and the loneliness experienced by the divorced husband and wife. It is not good for man to be alone and divorce results in loneliness. It is not good for children to be deserted by their parents, and divorce results in deserted children. It is unthinkable that God could have any other attitude to divorce. The message of Malachi is that God *hates* divorce. I know we all have our beliefs, but if I can keep anyone from experiencing what our family went through, God knows, I will be a witness. Don't come this way!

The message of Hosea is "reconciliation." If any separated couples are reading this book please reconsider. The prophet Hosea was called by God to live out his message to his people, by marrying a woman who would be unfaithful to him, and so his marriage was a symbolic picture of the relationship between God and his people. Hosea was to proclaim Israel's need for reconciliation to their faithful, loving God. The key verse is: The Lord said to me, 'Go, show your love to your wife again, though she is loved by another and is an adultress. Love her as the Lord loves the Israelites, though they turn to other gods' (Hosea 3: 1).

Hosea's wife had been unfaithful and committed adultery with other men. God saw her behavior as symbolic of the unfaithfulness of his people who were running after other gods, and being unfaithful to the covenant God had made with them. They promised to love Him with all their hearts, and to have no other gods. But they had been disloyal by worshipping man-made idols. Yet God did not cast them aside, even though they had betrayed him. Although He was angry and offended by their unfaithfulness and waywardness, He invited his people to return and repent of their sin. The Lord said, 'I will heal their waywardness and love them freely, for my anger has turned away from them' (Hosea 14:4). Despite their unfaithfulness, God was merciful and offered them the hope of reconciliation. In the same way as God acted towards faithless Israel, He directed Hosea to act towards his unfaithful wife, who was running after other men. Despite the fact that she was adulterous, God did not tell Hosea to divorce his wife, but rather to love her again. It is clear that God wanted Hosea to restore the relationship; He wanted Hosea to be reconciled, even though his wife was an adulteress, and the Law of Moses permitted him to divorce her. The question is – what is God saying to you?

In a study conducted by George Barna, a leading Christian research expert, divorce rates are highest among non-denominational Christian faith groups with Baptists denominational divorced couples following closely in second place. Barna uses the term "non-denominational" to refer to Evangelical Christian congregations that are not affiliated with a specific denomination. The vast majority are fundamentalist in their theological beliefs.

Children Divorce Statistics: Children divorce statistics give especially the skeptical people who do not accept anything as true, sound data as something to consider. These days most people accept divorce as a way of life, completely unaware of the damage they are doing to their children. Tell your friends, acquaintances and co-workers to read these shocking statistics about divorce and children. It may help them to reconsider divorce.

General children divorce statistics: 50% of all North-American children will witness the divorce of their parents.

Almost half of them will also see the breakup of a parent's second marriage. (Furstenberg and others -Life Course-)

One out of 10 children of divorce experiences three or more parental marriage breakups. (Gallagher, The Abolition of Marriage)

40% of children growing up in America today are being raised without their fathers. (Wade, Horn and Busy, Fathers, Marriage and Welfare Reform, Hudson Institute Executive Briefing, 1997)

50% of all the children born to married parents today will experience the divorce of their parents before they are 18 years old. (Fagan, Fitzgerald, Rector, the Effects of Divorce on America).

    Like never before I am so sure of my calling. I am called to be a helper of mankind. If I had never experienced a challenge and came out to be a witness, I would never be able to help others. I offer to you that now I know I am called to help people be clear about their call in life and to help restore, rebuild and reconcile families to trust God and live destiny! I have a dream to help others. I grew up in a single family home and now my children are experiencing the same thing. It's very clear that God wants me to take this mountain of family. What is God saying in this area? The first family He created in the beginning of time was the original family of Adam and Eve. How can we break this generational curse that has destroyed so many in this world, unless we come to a place of brokenness, and realize that nothing else matters except to be in the place that God has destined for us to be?

There must be more ministers, pastors, and intercessors that will be relentless in prayer and fasting; more teaching and equipping people from prior experiences and the Word of God. The manufacturer God himself wrote the manual for family. Until we – the product – go and seek his counsel on what to do in times of crisis, we will surely fail. I didn't like what happened to our family and so many others all over the world. There is absolutely nothing impossible for God. I can sulk about it or move on and say, *"I'm still here."* Now what can I do for my Father to demonstrate to Him and others I am still Created 2 Produce in this area? Forget those things which are behind, and press towards the mark. There is a mark and a prize that God wants each of us to attain in life after every challenge. I decided to move with God. It's my turning point and yours as well. More than anything my relationship with God grew in a measure that I can never explain. If I had never gone through it, I wouldn't be where I am today. Thank you Jesus for meeting me and others right where we are. How many can I help? How many impacts can I help birth in the spirit? I am here God. Send me. I'll go.

2 Peter 1:10: "Therefore, brethren, be even more diligent to make your call and election sure, for if you do these things you will never stumble." God wants us to be clear about our destiny and calling. It wasn't until I went through my challenges, that it became clear to me. There needs to be something within us that will not settle for less than what He has called us to. God planted the seeds of destiny in our hearts before we were born (Proverbs 4:23).

We grow and understand our destiny in the place of intimacy and communion with God. This is where we will discover our destiny determined before the foundation of the world. Does that sound crazy? The place where I will discover my destiny may be through divorce, lay off, foreclosure, and illness. I'm here to tell you miracles can happen if you are open to the voice of God. Open your mouth and repeat after me, *"God, What's Next?"*

Dr. Cassandra Scott is a true embodiment of a Woman of God. I've had the great fortune of knowing and being under her powerful, persuasive and Spirit-filled tutelage since 1998. Without reservations I know that she is my Spiritual Mother who has poured into me through word, seed and deed.

This Woman of God has been so very instrumental and impactful in my life. I've never had to look for her in my darkest hours, especially when my mother passed away. She's been very supportive. I often say that if the Bible was still in the process of being written, she would have a book within it. We read about Ruth, Naomi, Deborah, Sarah, Job, David and so on, which is fine, but she is a present-day living testimony of a Godly walk. I am not serving prison time now because of her walk and posture. She showed me how to go through an embarrassing divorce and allow God to handle the situation. During this time of great shaking she made sure that I purchased my 1st laptop, became computer literate and helped me realize that "Every girl needs a Plan B". She not only told me what to do during adverse times, but she showed me. She postured herself to help me while she was healing. I gained tremendous strength and respect for her, because she kept pressing.

As a result of her relentless tenacity she obtained her Associates, Bachelor's, Master's and Doctorate along with starting The Prayer line, Bible Study and from that Turning Point Faith Ministries. Dr. Scott offered no excuse not to continue on...she did it!

I'm grateful for her instilling in me that I was Created 2 Produce...life happens, but life is still what you make of it. She's challenged me, pushed me, prayed for me and supported me and told me about myself. I'm rough around the edges, but she keeps me around...loll. I will never forget the day that she called me and apologized after being convicted by a statement Bishop T.D. Jakes made, "Quit trying to change The Peters in your life. If Jesus kept His, you need to keep yours. They are anointed to do what they do". She calls me Peterine ~AKA~ ShugaThug.

Embrace yourself to benefit from the pen of this mighty woman of God,

Carol Smith

9

Prepare For A Miracle

No matter what you are experiencing in your life today! You can begin again. This is your turning point. The challenge will be: Do I keep pondering what should have, or could have, or do I move forward? I decided to move forward. There was so much more that God wanted me to see. As long as I wallowed in my sorrow, I could never see that I was Created 2 Produce. In all of the pain and shame, there was victory. I was expecting. Thank God I didn't abort the dream. Inside of me was something so great that I would have never imagined. Inside your greatest pain is the greatest miracle.

You will deliver. It's time to prepare. Isaiah 66:8 says, "Who has heard such a thing? Who has seen such things? Shall a land be born in one day? Shall a nation be brought forth in one moment? For as soon as Zion was in labor she brought forth her children."

My stomach was so big, my back hurt so bad, I could hardly breath, I couldn't sleep at night, I had to prop myself up on pillars just for comfort at night. I thought if I don't deliver this baby soon, I feel as if I could die. My feet and nose were swollen. I began to not look like myself. Some of you reading this book have changed drastically. You are so pregnant people

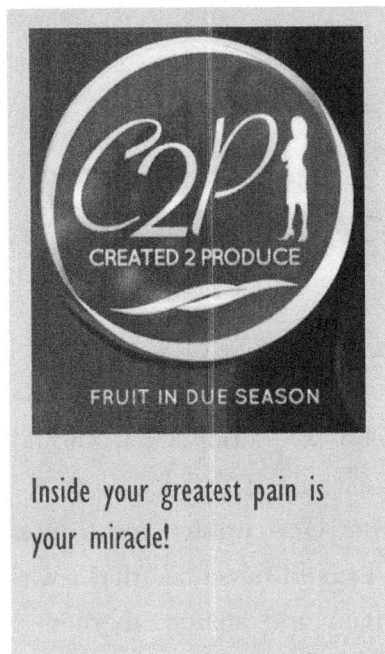

Inside your greatest pain is your miracle!

don't even recognize who you are. They can't understand why you don't fit with them anymore. You need to bust a move. When Abram was pregnant he had to move around. He wasn't even allowed to remain with his family. Can you imagine giving birth and your family is no where around? This miracle you are carrying is so big. It's in you but it's not really about you. I didn't care what I was having I just knew I needed to get it out of me. I couldn't move fast. I had a funny walk. My space was filled to capacity, I was so uncomfortable and it was not cute anymore. I had to take off my stilettos, I had to wear flats (ya'll know I don't like flats).

There were some events I just couldn't attend. It would be more trouble than what it was worth. This is where most men and women of God are. You will not even make it to full term. You will deliver within eight months or earlier, but your ministries will be healthy with no complications or ICU. God said, *"I have been grieved by your backaches from the largeness of your belly. You have carried my heavy desire these many months and indeed your back is weary."*

I can see Mary and Joseph going from one inn to another asking for somewhere to lay and deliver baby Jesus. Everywhere

Prepare For A Miracle

they went doors closed in their face but they were getting close to the place. Whatever you do, don't stop you are almost at the door that God has ordained for you to deliver your miracle. It didn't look like it and it didn't feel like it but Mary and Joseph were about to make a turning point in history. I wonder how people could be so cruel no you need them and close the door on you. It's all a part of the plan.

Many doors have been closed in your face. You have not been able to deliver where you thought naturally it made sense. God is preparing a barn for you to deliver and only those who He has invited will come to see your miracle in the beginning months! It's crucial for the life of your miracle. God will deliver you early from your pregnancy. God is inducing your womb and commanding you to produce his blessing.

I went to my doctor's appointment and she said prepare it's almost time. She said things like, *"Did you remember what we went over the day you found out you were pregnant? Things that needed to be prepared for the birth of the new born for this appointed day?"*

All three of my babies in the natural were delivered by C-Section. The doctor said I was too small to deliver and she didn't want the baby to go into fetal distress – so she would take the baby. She would induce the labor! Some of your babies are too big and your ministry will go into fetal distress if the Lord does not literally cut it out. Some will deliver vaginally and some by C-Section. Ready Yourself. Prepare to Deliver. You are Created 2 Produce.

Prepare for early delivery: I'm reminded while we sat in the waiting room, some women had early deliveries. They said, it's not even full term but my water has broken or I have started dilating. This is also a spiritually sign as well, the Holy Spirit is revealing early deliveries for many of His pregnant sons and daughters (literally). Many babies will not be carried to a full nine-month term. Many in the Body of Christ have been chosen to go into labor early, but still deliver healthy normal ministries, businesses, writing books, etc.

I was sitting in a service and suddenly was asked to speak and the word came forth without any strain. Many in the body of Christ will hold your beautiful blue eyed infant, nursing from your breast to become healthy and whole. Many will deliver this new thing early. God will reward you for your faithfulness; He will cut short your calculated pregnancy time that was originally recorded. You have waited long enough. Get Ready. It's Time. In physical pregnancy, when a woman/family is preparing for a new baby, there are roughly nine ways in which they prepare. I remember my to-do-list from my doctor. My doctor went over all these things with me nine months before the actual birth. These paralleled the preparations to be made for your new God-thing. Only you know what you are carrying inside you, so you and the Holy Spirit make the personal applications.

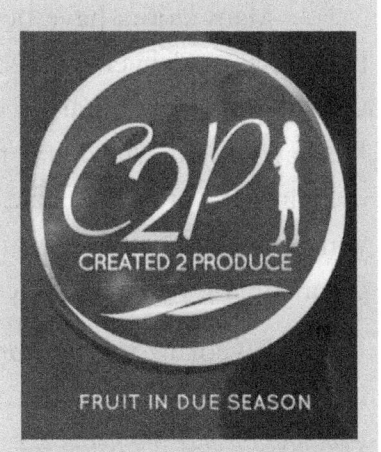
It's in you, but it's not really about you.

Your "To Do" List:

1. **Get your financial and legal affairs in order**: My spending habits had to drastically change. Babies come with new expenses and legalities. It's now not just about me, myself and I. Therefore expecting families modify their budget redirecting financial streams to baby-care supplies, savings, insurance policies, the establishment of wills, and so on.

   God's new thing will also come with new expenses and legalities. You would be surprised how many launch out into ministry and never count the cost. Waiting until it is finally here to make modifications will be too late. Worst case scenario, your baby could be aborted or put up for adoption (given to someone who did prepare, Mt 25:26-29). Best case scenario, you will have headaches and complications that could have been avoided completely. Get your financial and legal affairs in order.

2. **Stock the kitchen.** Nothing is worse than not having what you need when your baby is crying. A shrieking baby at 2 a.m. is not the best time to make a grocery run for Gerber or Huggies. Therefore, expecting families stock their kitchen with nutritional supplies well in advance.

   The new thing in Scripture: food is a symbol for knowledge and wisdom (Psalms 119:103, Proverbs 24:23, 14, Ezekiel 3:1-3, Hebrews 5:12-14, 1 Peter 2:2). Therefore, a kitchen would be akin to our mind, where we accumulate and store such intelligence. In fact, people often have dynamic dreams about their kitchen. Sometimes (not always), these dreams are revealing important information about mental contents and processes. In preparation for our new thing, we too have to stock our kitchen. Get rid of stuff you no longer need or that has expired. We will need pantries of new information and intelligence. You can't live on yesterday's manna, what is God saying today! We will need new proverbs and quotes to snack on. We might think we understand our new thing now, however, when it fully arrives, it will take on new meanings. Become an expert on your new thing before it appears. When faced with a situation, you need only to apply the information you've accumulated. Stock the kitchen. When it's your time to deliver you must release what has been stocked. Do you have anything in your kitchen pantry or is it empty or has nothing of nutritional substance?

3. **Baby-proof the house.** Our home was not baby-proof. Only adults had been living in our home for years. I read that expecting parents should realize the inside of their home can be hazardous. They put covers on sockets, fix or remove sharp edges, put small objects out of reach, rearrange furniture, and so on. The baby, though precious and lovable, knows nothing of safety. Who will hedge up the way and not be careless and let your baby put the first thing they see in their mouth? The new thing homes are perfect symbols for our lives. They are often the focus of our nightly dreams, indicating the condition of our life or

specific areas (rooms) of it. In preparation for the new thing, our lives must be updated and rearranged, primarily in the "little things" we tend to belittle or overlook. Song of Songs 2:15: Catch for us the foxes, the little foxes that ruin the vineyards, our vineyards that are in bloom. Sockets must be covered, the new thing should not have access to every aspect of our life; keep it in its place and proper perspective. Fix or remove sharp edges, rough or non-Christ like edges in our personality could harm the new thing; grow and change. What do you need to rearrange to ensure the baby's safe transplant into your life?

4. **Develop the nursery.** All of my children had different themes when they were born for their nursery. I ran all over the stores looking to decide which nursery décor I would choose. They were all simply beautiful. Before each of them were born, I would just go and sit in the nursery and rock in the chair and wonder what it would be like once I held the miracle from God. Expecting families develop a nursery for the baby, complete with a crib, rocking chair, baby imagery and decor, and other nursery-related supplies. Here, the baby sleeps and rests in cozy solitude. Sleep is crucial to the newborn's healthy development. One thing that I wanted to make sure was in the nursery was the monitor – so even thou I was not in the room – I could hear all that was going on. If they moved I could hear it. I got so behind on my daily work that I had to reorganize my days, because I was obsessed with every coo, cry or movement; running back and forth.

As a result, dinner, washing, and paying bills were going lack! I needed to get myself together! I got so overwhelmed and tired I would have to ask someone to come and get the baby or drop it off so I could go on with life on a daily basis as well. Your new thing will also need times of sleep. It will require regular periods of inactivity and disengagement. In other words, we cannot become obsessive or consumed by our new thing. We will need to simply "let it rest" and go about other activities, interests, and obligations. Don't lose yourself in your new thing. Prepare a nursery for it. It will need breaks from you and you will need breaks from it. In your ministry let someone else teach or preach for you and give yourself a break so you can miss it and it miss you.

5. **Prepare to travel.** Expecting parents prepare to travel with their little one. They purchase a federally-approved car seat, and in some cases, an entirely new vehicle. They prepare a "baby bag", stocked with diapers, a blanket or two, change of clothes, plastic bags, baby wipes, and other necessities. At one point my bag was so overloaded, I had to stop carrying my purse. I remember at one service our church was on program. After the benediction, the pastor of that church said on the microphone, "Excuse me everyone, but someone has lost their purse". I stood there and looked at the purse and then it clicked, that's my purse. I was too overwhelmed with all I had to carry once the baby was born. God loves experiencing new places through us and with us. This is the romantic side of Him. Ninety-nine percent of the time the new thing will take us

to new places, whether it is another part of the city or another part of the world. Get your car tuned up and ready or get a new one. Get your passport. Get a website. Get some business cards. Prepare your suitcases. Enhance your cell phone plan. Prepare to travel with your new baby. Doors were swinging open and I was going in. This time I wasn't alone because I had proof of what I had been carrying.

6. **Involve the siblings.** A new baby can arouse fiery reactions of jealousy in siblings. Therefore, expecting parents are encouraged to involve them in the preparation process. This refreshes their inclusion and value to the family, and, gives them personal contribution to the baby's arrival and welfare. Garelyn was the only child for almost five years before baby Gabrielle was born. I am so grateful that Garelyn was visited by angels in a dream months before I was even pregnant. She told us angels visited her and said we would have a baby sister! We looked in amazement as she told the story. So God got her little heart ready to receive and we made all the necessary arrangements to let her know she would still hold that special place in our hearts! It happened just like Garelyn's dream. A baby girl was born. Involve loved ones in your new thing preparations though not 100% foolproof, it greatly reduces the possibility of jealousy and resentment when the new thing appears. Remember, your new thing is not ultimately about you and your fulfillment. It is for God's public beauty and the saving of many lives (Gen 50:20). You may have delivered multiple ministries,

make sure you don't cause them to despise each other. Much prayer and great teams helping you will be the solution to cause spiritual siblings to not become jealous of each other.

7. **Seek childcare.** Expecting parents seek out child care, especially if Mom is going back to work. A great childcare situation might take time to arrange, so major attention is often applied here. Parents want to know their newborn is being cared for with the same passion they feel. Your new thing will require childcare. God does not intend for you to manage it all alone, at least not permanently or as a rule. We would exhaust ourselves, and possibly harm the baby. He always sends a friend and babysitter. Saul had Samuel. David had Jonathan. Elijah had Elisha. Paul had a small team. Even Jesus' messianic ministry had childcare--twelve disciples. There is someone(s) around you providentially positioned to help you manage your new thing. Let them care for your blessing while you rest and tend to other matters.

Who will be your baby's spiritual god parents or baby sitters? Who are the people that you can trust to keep your baby for you without stealing it once it's born? God blessed our children to have wonderful grandparents: Edwin and Naomi Hilliard, Pastor Ollie and Doris Scott and wonderful God parents: Brother Frank and Alyce Kinney, Pastor Tim and Stephanie Glynn and Sadie Jackson. They also had wonderful aunts and uncle. We never had to worry about them stealing the miracles He gave us. Not only were they in their lives as babies, but still today, speaking and sowing wisdom and a strong support system as ordained by God.

A Word of Wisdom

You need someone who will speak life into your gift, not just someone who will buy them a lot of clothes, baby sit, or come to a birthday party once a year. You need someone who will impart wisdom and knowledge into the lives ordained by God. When you have your baby naturally or spiritually – who will you trust with your child?

2 Samuel 4:4 (Jonathan son of Saul had a son who was lame in both feet. He was five years (5 number of grace) old when the news about Saul and Jonathan came from Jezreel. His nurse picked him up and fled, but as she hurried to leave, he fell and became crippled. His name was Mephibosheth.) 2 Samuel 9 David asked, "Is there anyone still left of the house of Saul to whom I can show kindness for Jonathan's sake?"So Mephibosheth ate at David's table like one of the king's sons.

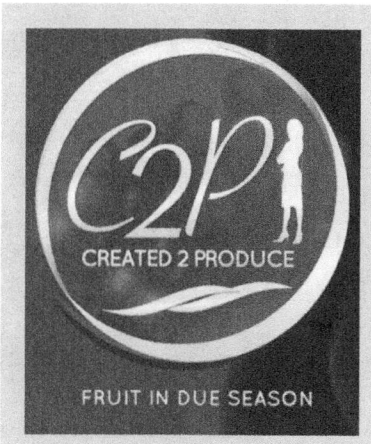

Some of you have been dropped by your parents, spouse, family and friends, spiritual fathers and mothers.

Remember Mephibosheth?

His nurse dropped him when he was only five years old and he was crippled the rest of his life. Will the person you have entrusted with your baby drop it? I've been dropped, what about you? Guess what? Even if you or your ministry has been dropped the King is waiting for you! Some of you have been dropped by your parents, spouse, family and friends, spiritual fathers and mothers. They never came back to get you.

You have looked out the window long enough. They are not coming back. God has assigned someone else to pick you up. Have you ever felt like you were all alone or in a desert place? I feel your hurt and your pain but God will remind your David of the promise He made to Jonathan, David and his family will not forget about you. No one can eat or proceed with the party or celebration until you get to the table. No matter how long it takes you to get there. You may come dragging your foot, on crutches, in a wheel chair, or even a stretcher. But I prophesy you will get to your destination! You are Created 2 Produce!

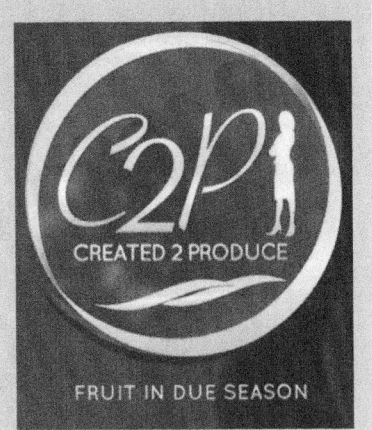

Lord, I am not worthy to receive you, only say the words and I shall be healed. Luke 7: 6

You have looked out the window long enough. They are not coming back...You will get to your destination.

And when they could not bring him to Jesus because of the crowd, they removed the roof above him; these four friends were ingenious and persistent. They were going to find a way to get their sick buddy in front of Jesus the healer. They didn't let a crowd stop them like the brother in the Bible carried by his four friends. God will interrupt the church service and allow your friends to take the roof off the house and lower you down in the front of the service to get your healing and deliverance and publicly start your ministry. All eyes shall see you spring forth. The promise is yours.

I'm reminded of so many of my friends that saw me paralyzed. They would come to my house and pray for me. I couldn't even pray for myself. They literally carried me into the presence of God. Women like Naomi Hilliard, Carol Smith, Tongela Clark, Apostle Jacqueline Phelps, Alyce Kinney, Gloria Archie, Martha Hardin, Pastor Liddie Owens, Pastor Eleanor Murray, Stephanie Glynn, Stephanie King, Dorthy Fields and so many more. They knew that I was pregnant with greatness and cared enough for me in my weakest hour to lower me in the presence of the Lord. They didn't talk about me or criticize me. They prayed for me. They backed up in my tent and literally covered me up like Noah sons did in the Bible. Do you have any friends like that? Or do you have friends that are jealous of what you are carrying and can't wait till you die so they can illegally take your ministry, husband or wife, job or children and friends and act as if it were their dream or idea. I don't like baby snatchers. Watch out for them they are all around.

8. **Find a good physician**. Expectant mothers need a good physician, one that is medically proficient and one the mother feels comfortable being naked in front of. Are you comfortable enough to take off your clothes in front of your doctor? If not, you better keep looking, because my doctor saw everything. The good, the bad and the ugly; she saw all of the stretch marks, hemorrhoids, etc.

9. **Don't lose touch with the baby's father**. Tragically, many mothers lose touch with the very man who fathered their baby. When possible, wise mothers must take care to keep intimate touch with the father. If not, fathers have been known to resent the newborn and the mother. In extreme cases, jealous fathers can resort to cheating, domestic abuse, and even infanticide. Thank God for your baby daddy. Imagine how Joseph felt when Mary told him she was pregnant. He wasn't there during the conception and was now he was expected to help take care of a child that was supposed to be from God? He had to hear from God to not get in the way of Jesus being birth.

The new thing: Pregnant Christians don't lose touch with the Father. He impregnated you with this wonderful new thing. He cared for you throughout the difficult preparation process. He kept you sane when your pregnancy was misunderstood and persecuted. And now, you are only moments away from delivering the blessing.

Don't stop spending that alone time romancing Him. Don't stop pleasuring Him in worship. Don't stop cuddling with Him and holding His hand. Don't lose touch with the Everlasting Father. Like a jealous earthly father our heavenly Father has been known to resent even destroy the very new thing He created if the human caretakers demote Him. Remember the many revivals and movements that came and ended miserably. Remember the Flood. Remember David and Bathsheba's first baby. Remember the exodus generation slain in the desert. Hosea 9:11-14. *11 Ephraim's glory will fly away like a bird-- no birth, no pregnancy, and no conception. 12 Even if they rear children, I will bereave them of every one. Woe to them when I turn away from them! 13 I have seen Ephraim, like Tyre, planted in a pleasant place. But Ephraim will bring out their children to the slayer. "14 Give them, O LORD—what will you give them? Give them wombs that miscarry and breasts that are dry.*

Don't lose touch with the Father and provoke His jealousy by putting more emphasis on the birth than the birth giver. He is a jealous God and will not have any other God before Him. I've seen so many people get that special gift from God and then forget all about Him; the God who made it possible. No more praying, fasting, and submitting, because the gift has been misplaced and caused you to get off focus of the true purpose.

Deliver the Miracle

When I look back from all of the pain, I was able to deliver miracles and hidden treasures that I never knew were inside of me. I was able to name each of my babies naturally and now spiritually. I never knew I was pregnant with:

Cassandra Scott Ministries (CSM) Bible Study in home – (started with my three children and it grew into a church, Turning Point Faith Ministries – birthed in August 2009 and presently pastoring over 40 families);

CSM Prayer line – birthed in May 2010 with 20 members of Turning Point Faith and now praying for over 200 people daily every morning on a 6am prayer line; 13 directors are now rotating weekly in prayer and focuses to build and equip intercessors in prayer;

CSM Mentorship – yearly 6 month mentorship for men and women to discover who they are in Christ; equipping in the five-fold ministry gifts; helping to produce God-given assignments;

CSM International Prayer Summit – held annually May of each year. Intercessors all over the world attend to be equipped for ministry;

CSM Regional Seminars/Workshops – 2013 preparing to go to different states to help people understand that you are to trust God and live destiny.

The Book, Created 2 Produce - Now, I am releasing my first book. This book will be used to open other doors all over the world. We will provide workshops, seminars and conferences to help people realize they are Created 2 Produce.

Pastor Cassandra Scott is true to her namesake of helper of mankind. She has been my First Lady, Pastor, friend, and physical and spiritual birth coach for more than 15 years - during some of the most pivotal years of my life. Because of the call of God upon her life, I now have two sons, Bishop and Elisha Ray who were born after two miscarriages and a series of pregnancy complications. I was one of the women she first laid hands on in the Fruitful Womb Ministry to conceive. Not only did we have one son after she prayed with us, we had two, when before – all we had were miscarriages and tears.

The presence of God lingered upon us for years through the anointing that follows the life of Pastor C with signs and wonders. Through her prayer ministry, I fell in love with God, developed a real relationship with the Holy Spirit, and learned to love my life in Jesus Christ with a passion that has never grown old.

I will never forget the time when the prayer that she and her husband prayed for me and my family, saved our lives and kept us from a dangerous assignment that had been dispatched from the enemy.

In January 2000, by the laying on of hands and through the transference of the anointing that was upon her, God manifested Himself to me for the first time through tongues and the Holy Spirit's prayer language at the very first women's retreat that she participated in while we were at Trinity Fellowship Houston. It was a night that I would never forget, and one that I often draw new strength, revelation, and glory from today because the hands of Jesus touched me in a whole new way. I will always thank God for Pastor C and Bishop G for sharing the Gospel of Jesus Christ with me, watching out for my life, building my family, and propelling me toward the bright destiny God purposed for me and my family. –Blessings galore!

Merle Ray

10

God's Got This

I was called from the womb. God set His hand on me from the beginning. He separated me and set me apart. I've always felt separated. I never really fit in. It seems people didn't really receive me while growing up and as an adult. I've noticed sometimes I live a lonely life. If you trace the life of an apostle, I fit the description. In Galatians 1:15 Paul says: But when it pleased God, who set me apart from my mother's womb, and called [me] by his grace, 16 to reveal his Son in me, that I might preach him among the gentiles.

You have also been called from the womb. You were Created 2 Produce. It pleases God to know that you and I are separated for Him. Your whole life has been a preparation. Your preparation began when the seed met the egg. When the sperm and egg joined together in your mother's womb the calling was there already. God knew you. When Jesus hung on the cross He looked down, He saw you, and He knew you. And He ordained you and you were set apart unto the gospel of God, unto the call of God. You were chosen and you were called. You were given a mandate. Take the mantle.

Even though I was separated and set a part, I would always wonder? Why in ministry they prophesy better, at school they got a higher grade and in business they got the deal that I could not close. How could they take my notes and excel pass me? The Christian thing to do would be to "just walk in love". But let's get real here. It hits you and me in the gut and frustrates the life out of you. You always wonder why you seem to keep falling short of the mark. That question always haunted me. You start asking questions like, *"What is wrong with me?"* or *"What makes them so special?"* I would always find myself asking questions like, *why couldn't I have stay married? Why can't I lose weight? Why did I have difficulty in conceiving spiritually and naturally? Why don't people accept me?* Do you know what the problem is with this kind of questioning? You end up messing up the opportunities that God really does want to give you, and the worst of it is you slowly lose the lust for life.

Well today I am here to help bring your joy back. The Lord has a special place for you and all that you need to do now is to take your eyes off what everyone else is doing, and focus on what God has given you to do.

I am going to help you out a bit here. Look at these questions and answer them for yourself:

- What calling or responsibility has God given to you?
- What did you do today towards this call?

Whether you are called to ministry, holding down a regular job, in charge of a business, or your family, you have a place and until you excel in it, you cannot stop to look at what everyone else is doing. There is a danger when you do that. You start to compare yourself to others. In fact you get so busy looking at what everyone else is doing that you do not flow in the gifts and anointing God has given to you. You forget that it is the Lord that has said it and would do it. The next thing you know the anointing has lifted and you find yourself wandering the desert for a couple of years.

Just like the twelve spies that spied out the land, ten had an evil report (UNBELIEF) and two had a good report (FAITH). There will always be two voices speaking at the border of your breakthrough, determine to listen and listen again and follow the voice of faith.

I found myself like the ten, always focusing on my flesh. I was in church hearing the word, shouting all over the church, believing for everyone else but myself, prophesying for everyone else, and I had a spirit of unbelief when it came to me. Because of unbelief we miss the opportunity of the Promise Land. We are right at the border and then talk ourselves right out of the deal. The hurting thing is not only do you miss the promise but those who are following or connected to you get thrown off as well. My mind needed to be renewed by the Word of God.

It is time to focus 100% on what God has given you. The good news is that what God has given to you is unique. He has called you and He has every intention on helping you follow through. I asked the question like Mary. *How can I do this? How can I start a ministry? How can I raise my children as a single parent? How can I pastor a church as a woman? How can I mentor others and equip them for the work of ministry? How can I raise up leaders in business and* ministry, *How can I? How can I? How can I?* God spoke to me and said, *"You can't, but I can. I will send you a helper who will come on you and the power of the Most High will overshadow you."* Not only did He speak these wonderful words to me, He connected me to men and women who where carriers of the wonderful hidden treasures of heaven that would understand me and mentor and coach me through. He will do the same for you. You are not alone.

I finally said, "Your will be done in my life." I let go and stopped trying to be in charge. I don't understand it all, normally He shows me little by little just testing if I will trust him for the victory each step of the way. God has the complete plan all worked out. Repeat after me: Be it unto me, according to your words. May your words be fulfilled. This is your turning point.

"How will this be," Mary asked the angel, "since I am a virgin?" 35 The angel answered, "The Holy Spirit will come on you, and the power of the Most High will overshadow you, so the holy one to be born will be called the Son of God. 36 Even Elizabeth your relative is going to have a child in her old age, and she who was said to be unable to conceive is in her sixth month. 37 For no word from God will ever fail." 38 "I am the Lord's servant," Mary answered. "May your word to me be fulfilled?" Then the angel left her.

I came from a generation of believers of God. I was born into this call. I have known the Lord all of my life. I grew in the knowledge in the Lord. I grew up witnessing and sharing. I was different. I had very few friends. My whole life, I had a passion for the Lord.

In the sixth grade I told all of my classmates of the coming of the Lord. I had great plans to work in corporate America, but in the middle of those plans God changed everything for me. I developed a career in oil and gas industry. The leader of church said I would marry a minister; I thought how in the world? I would always go back and forth in business and ministry. I have been chosen to lead God's people out of the Egypts of this world.

My assignment is clear. I flow in the five fold ministry gifts. I have been chosen by God to train and equip leaders in family, business and ministry. I've been sent to help men, women boys and girls to discover or produce what God has inside of them.

One day I met my friend Tongela Clark for lunch. I parked my car and waited for her to pick me up. When she drove up she let her window down and said, "Come on and get in". I got my purse, locked my car door and proceeded to get in her car. She said in a loud voice, "Get in preacher".

Immediately, the next words I heard in her car stereo were, "I've got this," which are the words to a song by Jennifer Hudson. I had never heard it before. My faith was stirred, my spirit leaped and the preacher in me got one of the best sermons I ever preached. Immediately God spoke those words to me and it has been with me since then. God's Got This. I don't care who you are, what you are going through. God's Got This.

Reflecting on what God has already done helps us anticipate what He is about to do. Remember what God has done for you. Think of the times when He delivered you.

Rehearse the miracles He brought to pass in your life. Recall God's miraculous provisions. Your memories of what God has done can release your faith in God to do it again.

"Reflection" is remembering what God has done. "Anticipation" is realizing He will do it again. As I jotted down some of the things that came to my mind as a reflection of God's miraculous provision, He gave me a turning point miracle in each of these customized testimonies. *Ain't no stopping me.* I keep growing. I will reach each goal. Put your hand in the air if you know God's Got This. All of these things were necessary to shape my character into the very image of God. It was a process and preparation for my calling. Look at my list of trials and/or challenges that are now customized testimonies:

- I didn't know who I was as a person with identity issues and low self esteem as a child and adult.
- I didn't know who I was as a former pastor's wife.
- Married for 21 years and went through a divorce in 2007. I was embarrassed and ashamed after the divorce; I could hardly look people in their eyes because of the tormenting spirits that called me a failure 24/7.
- Growing up in a single family home. Raised on welfare. Sitting and looking out the window at other families. Longing for the same for my life.
- Unable to have children in 1986-87.
- My faith, family, finances and future were under attack by the enemy after divorce.

- My father had a major heart attack and was pronounced dead for 20 minutes in 2010.
- In 2011 my mother was in ICU at St Luke's Hospital and my dad was in ICU at Hermann Hospital *at the same time for weeks*. My brothers and I running from one hospital to the oth*er and I still had a mind* to serve God.
- My mother went home to be with the Lord in 2011, and she was with me every step of the way whether I failed or succeeded. God gave me strength to preach her homegoing service.
- Fear of starting my own church in August 2009 as a single mother and woman in ministry.
- Obeyed God in May 2010 and started a weekly prayer line. It grew from 20 members of Turning Point Faith Ministries into an international prayer ministry. We are ministering and praying for over 1000 people weekly. Thirteen directors rotate weekly to equip and train intercessors in prayer.

Selah!

God has given me victory in every area of my life. When I think about the goodness of Jesus and all He has done for me, I could dance, dance, dance all night.

I came to give you hope in the message that He will do it again. Not one of the trials that I went through is a situation that I can't find in the Word of God. God's Got This. God is not a one night wonder. A one night wonder is somebody who records a great song but you never hear from them again. A one night wonder is somebody who has a great professional ball game but never repeats that performance. A one wonder is somebody who writes a great book but never surfaces again. I have news for you. God is not a one night wonder.

Do a background check on God. You'll soon find that whatever He does once, He will always do again … and again … and again … and again … and again. God wants us to look back at what He has already done to create anticipation and release our faith that He will do it again. Here is a powerful formula.

REFLECTION + ANTICIPATION = MANIFESTATION

Think about the story of Abraham. Romans 4:19 tells us that Abraham considered his own body dead. He was 100 years old; as far as having a baby goes he was dead. Sarah's womb was also dead. Do you have anything that looks dead in your life right now? But Abraham did not waiver in his confidence in the promise of God that he would be the father of a great nation. In spite of the fact that their bodies were dead, Isaac was born. God raised the dead back to life. Get ready; God is about to raise something that has been dead in your life.

When God asked Abraham to sacrifice Isaac, he was confident because he knew that God brings the dead back to life. And he knew He would do it again. The Bible is filled with examples of how God's Got This. If you search you will see that miracle after miracle occurred multiple times in scripture. From Enoch to Moses to Joshua to Elijah to Jesus, each of them experienced God's miracle power repeatedly in their lives. He never did anything just once. Whatever God did once, He always did again.

So whatever you need in your life right now, find it one time in the Bible, and expect God to do it again. I feel a shout coming on. Someone reading this book is getting the revelation that God's Got This!

God parted the Red Sea for Moses – God parted the Jordan River for Joshua. Jesus multiplied five loaves and two fish – A few chapters later He did it again.

Enoch was caught up into the presence of God (Genesis 5) – Elijah went up in a to heaven (2 Kings 2:11) – Jesus ascended into heaven (Acts 1:11)

What do you need in your life right now? Do you need healing in your body? He has done that before. Do you need a blessing in your finances? Do you need a breakthrough in a relationship? Do you need God to restore some area of your life? He has done all that before; and if God has done something once, He will do it again. God wants to release His resurrection power in your life today.

Consider this: When you plant a seed in the ground, it dies to you and you die to it. But, you plant the seed knowing there will be a resurrection and when the seed dies, it produces an abundant harvest whose worth far exceeds the original seed. So when you plant a faith seed you release God's resurrection power in your life.

I planted faith seeds on all of the trials that I was going through. I practiced this night and day. It was my workout routine. I believed and I received when I prayed (Mark 9:2). I believed God is no respecter of persons (Romans 2:11). I believed in Biblical meditation (Joshua 1:8 and Ephesians 3:20). I was able to produce each of these miracles with the seed of God's Word through a simple process: meditation produces manifestation.

All my life it was so hard to believe because of my natural circumstances. I had to be renewed in my mind with the Word of God. It was a daily fight and still is. I had to realize that I was created in the very image of God. Did you hear me? I said, "The very image of God." I didn't make this up. I found it in the Word of God. I meditated on it daily while going through the storms of life.

It is written is the language you have to use on the enemy! I had to actually stand in the middle of my floor and say, "I am created in the very image of God." This information I found from the Christian Apologetics and Research Ministry website at www.Carm.org was helpful in understanding more about being made in the image of God.

The term "Image of God" occurs three times in the Bible. In Genesis 1:26-27 and 9:6, we find out that man is created in the image of God. In 2 Corinthians 4:4 we see the phrase used in reference to Jesus who is the "Image of God". There is no exact understanding of what the phrase means but we can generalize. It would seem that the first two verses refer to God's character and attributes that are reflected in people. The term cannot be a reference to a physical appearance of God since Jesus says in John 4:24 that God is Spirit, and in Luke 24:39 Spirit does not have flesh and bones. Therefore, we can conclude that the image of God deals with humanity's reflection of God in such things as compassion, rationality, love, hatred, fellowship, etc. God exhibits all of these characteristics, as do people. The Bible says that we are made in God's image. Genesis 1:26-27 - Then God said, "Let us make man in our image, in our likeness, and let them rule over the fish of the sea and the birds of the air, over the livestock, over all the earth, and over all the creatures that move along the ground." 27 So God created man in his own image, in the image of God he created him; male and female he created them.

When I became a Christian and read about being made in the image of God I wasn't sure what it actually meant. This tells me that God has hard wired His good things into my DNA. I may sin and fall short at times, but my DNA is firmly rooted, established and founded in Him. This passage gave me hope that my mom and dad were used by God to get me into the earth; we were purposed to live in the neighborhood we lived in, work at the jobs that hired us, and go to the churches that we connected to. It was all in the plan of preparation for purpose.

Just like Mary and Joseph were used to get Jesus here in the earth. He is a God of order and He would not illegally come into this world or kingdom of darkness without using a body, a member of the Body of Christ to bring light into that dark environment. I am part of the Most High God, the King and Creator of the universe.

This changed my thoughts now of how I was raised in a single family home etc. God used these things so that I could be a witness to others that have traveled down the same road. God knows He can trust you to have victory in those things that are pressing you right now.

The Bible says that we are no longer condemned. Romans 8:1 says, "Therefore, there is now no condemnation for those who are in Christ Jesus. One of my biggest faults as a new Christian was self condemnation. It was a pattern I was stuck in and I just couldn't shake it. If I did something wrong, I would beat myself up for days and sometimes even weeks. I used to talk to myself and say things like, "You call yourself a Christian and you did this again." I was destroying myself with destructive words.

I spoke without thinking. That cost me dearly. I was the type of person who had to have the last word. Because of this negative self talk, I was living way below where God wanted me to be. I was hamstrung because most of the time I walked around feeling condemned or that I didn't equal to others. I felt so low. I felt others always had it better than me. Whining me, myself, and I - I wasn't free. I am short 4 ft 11 in. I would dread when people would laugh at my height. I felt so worthless. I wasn't free as it talks about in John 8:36 (If the Son sets you free, you will be free indeed). Then one day God really spoke to my heart about it from Romans 8. Verses 33-34 say, *"Who dares accuse us whom God has chosen for His own? No one—for God himself has given us right standing with himself. Who then will condemn us? No one—for Christ Jesus died for us and was raised to life for us, and he is sitting in the place of honor at God's right hand, pleading for us"* (NLT).

I finally realized that if God the Father has declared me right with Himself and Jesus was always pleading my case before

Him, then I am not condemned. I am free from all condemnation—really, really truly free. I also realized that when I condemn myself, I am not following what God says about me in His Word. He has declared me righteous in His sight. Who am I to speak against God? The Bible says that I am free of all condemnation. You are free of all condemnation.

The Bible says that we are God's masterpiece. Ephesians 2:10 - For we are God's workmanship, created in Christ Jesus to do good works, which God prepared in advance for us to do. (NIV). The NLT uses the "Masterpiece" instead of workmanship. I really like that thought. God being the master craftsmen and He made me. Just like Michel Angelo painting the roof of the Sistine Chapel, God lovingly knit me together in my mother's womb. Psalm 139:13-14 echoes this thought. It says, "For you created my inmost being; you knit me together in my mother's womb. I praise you because I am fearfully and wonderfully made. Your works are wonderful, I know that full well." God made me and I am wonderfully made.

The other great thing about this passage is that I am here for a purpose. As I keep telling my children, we could have been born at any time in history, but God chose for us to live now. He made us with certain gifts and certain abilities to do certain things in this time and place. He has a plan and purpose for my life. I find this very exciting. I find this empowering. I find that this changes the way I see myself. I am not an afterthought. I am not a mistake. I am not a chance of evolution. I am a before thought. God had me on His mind before the foundations of the world.

God had you on His mind too. The Bible says that I am God's masterpiece. You are God's masterpiece too.

The Bible says that we are seated with Christ. Where you are seated at a special occasion often determines how important you are to the host of the function. If you are the bridal table at a wedding reception it means you are very special to the bride and groom.

If you are at the King's or Prime Minister's table at a special function you are held in very high regard. I was at Holy Convocation with Bishop Corletta Vaughn of Detroit, MI. I was seated in the audience and I was praising and blessing the Lord. Suddenly, one of the ushers tapped me on the shoulder and said, "Will you please follow me? Your name has been requested to sit on the podium with the Bishop." I looked up and saw all of the generals who had spoke at the meeting on the podium and I thought, *there is a seat for me?*

No matter who has taken your seat in the natural, you are seated spiritually at the right hand of the Father. Remember Joseph. It's a matter of time through preparation; you just have to make a couple of stops:

1) The pit,

2) The prison

3) The palace.

The devil in hell can't stop you from getting to your ultimate destination. Say with me, "I have a couple of stops to make but the end of the matter is better than the beginning." *Jesus! I feel the Holy Ghost.*

The Bible tells us that when Jesus returned to heaven He was seated at the right hand of the Father. That is the highest place of honor in the whole universe. There is no greater place than being seated next to the Father.

But that is not where the great news stops. You are also seated with Christ. Go ahead right now straighten out your royal robe and fix your crown on your head. It's leaning from some of the storms of life but it's still on your head. Let's have a look at what the Bible says in Ephesians Chapter 2:

But because of his great love for us, God, who is rich in mercy, made us alive with Christ, even when we were dead in transgressions—it is by grace you have been saved. And God raised us up with Christ, and seated us with him in the heavenly realms in Christ Jesus, in order that in the coming ages, he might show the incomparable riches of his grace, expressed in his kindness to us in Christ Jesus. (Ephesians 2:4-7 NIV)

If you are in Christ Jesus (that means in relationship with Him, trusting Him for your salvation, and have received Him as your King) then you are spiritually seated with Christ in the heavenly realms! You are spiritually seated with Him in the highest place in the universe. I will just let you soak that in a bit. You are Created 2 Produce!

Because of this great news you no longer have to walk around with your face pointing to the ground or your shoulders hunched over. You and I no longer have to feel unworthy. As a child and adult – I felt unworthy. We have high standing and high honor with the King and Creator of the universe. You and I are seated with Christ. The Bible says that I am seated with Christ in the heavenly realm. You are seated with God. He will give you peace

In His final days on earth, Jesus spoke at great lengths to His followers about the days to come. In John 16:33, He told them, "I have told you these things, so that in me you may have peace. In this world you will have trouble. But take heart! I have overcome the world."

This scripture jumped off the pages to me. I'm from another kingdom. What happens to me in this world has already been revealed to me from my Father. Growing up in a single family home, getting a divorce, having a miscarriage, getting into debt, fear of being alone, etc. God says, *"Take heart – I have overcome the World"*

As long as we live on this earth, we will have trouble. There will be days of shaking ahead. But the voice of Jesus gives us peace. He wants us to know that even though there is trouble all around us we belong to the One who has overcome the world. We are His children and He wants to carry us on His shoulders.

Peace is something we all need. When catastrophes strike, we need peace. When the economy fails, we need peace. When we face an uncertain future, we need peace. When everyone around us is fearful, we need peace. Jesus said in Luke 21 that men's hearts would fail them from fear and expectation of the things that were coming on the earth. Fear, anxiety, stress, and sorrow will overcome many. But for those who know their Father, who are lifted up and carried in His arms, there is nothing to fear. This peace that I have today the world didn't give it. I come as a witness you can be in the midst of the lion's dean and sleep in the fire.

You have victory. It is written.

Don't let your emotions take control: Meditate on the Word of God and believe it and receive the total victory that has already been paid. Some of the Scriptures I stood on and confessed daily were: Revelation 12:11; 1 John 5:3-5; Revelation 3:21; James 4:10; 1 Peter 5:8-10; 1 John 2:12-15; Deuteronomy 1:21; Deuteronomy 20:4; Psalm 44:6-8; Isaiah 26:3; Matthew 11:28; Mark 14:38; Romans 8:28; Romans 8:35.37; Romans 12:21; Colossians 3:10; Isaiah 43:7; Galatians 6:15; Ephesians 1:4; Ephesians 2:6; Ephesians 2:13; Jeremiah 29: 11; and Exodus 9: 16 – just to list a few.

My assignment is clear: I have an apostolic call on my life. I am an apostle. I operate in all of the five fold ministry gifts. I have been chosen by God to train and equip leaders for the work of ministry not just in church but in the area of business as well. I am to raise up as many leaders as God has assigned to my hands in faith, family, finances and futures. I've been sent to help men, women boys and girls to discover or produce what God has inside of them. This is your turning point Cassandra; you are a helper of mankind!

11

Winning The Battle Of The Mind

One day I was driving in my neighborhood, my easy access way; when I approached the road that I was to turn on I saw a sign and it said under construction, road closed, and detour. I got so mad because I had to go the long way around. That road was closed.

God then spoke to me saying, "This is what I need you to do regarding the enemy building or having access in your life on a daily basis through your thoughts." He has had easy access into these areas in your life, low self esteem, self righteousness, bitterness, depression, and all other kinds of negativity. He then can determine the outcome of your destiny, if you don't bring every thought that exalts itself against the knowledge of God or the truth of God's word into captivity.

I said, "What do you mean?" God said close those thoughts in your life that do not line up with my Word. These are areas that you have worried about morning, noon and night. Put a road block up today. Don't give the enemy access to keep traveling illegally in your mindset. I need you to meditate on my Word both day and night, so when the enemy comes, you will recognize if you need to navigate your thoughts. I want to give you victory in your mind.

Ephesians 6:10-11 – Finally my brethren, be strong in the Lord and in the power of his might. Put on the whole armor of God that you may be able to stand against the wiles of the devil.

According to the Hebrew-Greek dictionary, the word "wiles" in this verse could be translated as "schemes" or "methods." The word "wiles" comes from a Greek word "methodos," which means the devil has a method or a roadway to get into our lives.

Scheme: 1. a plan, design, or program of action to be followed; project. 2. An underhand plot; intrigue. 3. A visionary or impractical project. 4. A body or system of related doctrines, theories, etc.: a scheme of philosophy. 5. Any system of correlated things, parts, etc., or the manner of its arrangement.

Method: 1. a procedure, technique, or way of doing something, especially in accordance with a definite plan: There are three possible methods of repairing this motor. 2. A manner or mode of procedure, especially an orderly, logical, or systematic way of instruction, inquiry, investigation, experiment, presentation, etc.: the empirical method of inquiry. 3. An order or system in doing anything: to work with method. 4. An orderly or systematic arrangement, sequence, or the like.

We get the word "road" from the second part of this Greek word "odos". So when He says that the devil has a "wile" or a "method," what He is literally saying is that the devil has a method of building a road into your life so that once he gets access through that road, he can influence the outcome of your life. God tells us to "put on the whole armor of God that we may be able to stand against the wiles of the devil."

The devil has a scheme or a method to build a road and gain access into our lives. What is that road? As we see throughout the Bible, it is our thought life. Our thought life is the road Satan uses to drive into our finances, faith, families, marriage, health, and every other area of our lives. As we win the battle of our mind, we will experience the true freedom and power that we all long for. We do know that Satan does not have authority in our lives; but he deceives us with thoughts and lies so that once those thoughts get into our head, it paves the way for us to fall under his influence.

If you've ever experienced broken relationships, disappointing outcomes, moral failures, identity crisis, loss of a dream, or a divided family, I want to encourage you today. You have come to your turning point.

I have said for the last five years, *"Lord, when is my past going to stop influencing my present? Are you big enough to give me back what I've lost? Because I've tried it in my own strength, and it's not working."* What I have learned on my journey to wholeness is one touch from God in your life can change everything. He can do more in one moment than you can do in 20 years. I thought, "Oh My God", I was married for twenty years and we had nothing and we built a strong ministry, helped people all over the world. We lived in the largest homes, drove the finest cars, and had money in our bank account; we had no worries. Now I'm divorced, a single parent, business owner, pastor, and life coach; completed my doctorate in theology. *Why do I have to start all over? How can I do this alone?* God dealt with me like I imagined that He dealt with Mary *(I'll discuss in chapter 13).*

God has also given us wonderful instruction through Scripture about renewing our mind.

Some Benefits of Renewing Your Mind

1. **Renewing your mind transforms you.**

Romans 12:1-2 "I beseech you therefore, brethren, by the mercies of God, that ye present your bodies a living sacrifice, holy, acceptable unto God, which is your reasonable service. And be not conformed to this world: but, be ye transformed by the renewing of your mind, that ye may prove what is that good, and acceptable, and perfect, will of God."

We need to see ourselves like God sees us. Don't let your failures determine who you are, but let your determination be a reflection of God in your life. Look at yourself in the mirror of the Word of God.

2. **Renewing your mind makes you fruitful.**

Psalms 1:1-3

"Blessed is the man that walketh not in the counsel of the ungodly, nor standeth in the way of sinners, nor sitteth in the seat of the scornful. But his delight is in the law of the LORD; and in his law doth he meditate day and night. And he shall be like a tree planted by the rivers of water, that bringeth forth his fruit in his season; his leaf also shall not wither; and whatsoever he doeth shall prosper."

Bill Winston Ministries of Oak Park, Illinois shares that biblical meditation is a good thing. It is a God-given process that causes a permanent change in your thinking. The Bible declares: As a man thinketh in his heart so is he; in other words, *"What he believes is where he will end up."*

Joshua 1:8

"This book of the law shall not depart out of thy mouth; but thou shalt meditate therein day and night, that thou mayest observe to do according to all that is written therein: for then thou shalt make thy way prosperous, and then thou shalt have good success."

In Joshua 1:8, prosperity is tied to meditation. Also success is tied to meditation. God has done His part; now it is left up to you. Meditate means "to mutter or muse; to speak to oneself," and "to ponder the Word." You have to think bigger. Then you will be able to possess it and believe it.

3. Renewing your mind gives you peace.

Jeremiah 17:8

"For he shall be as a tree planted by the waters and that spreadeth out her roots by the river, and shall not see when heat cometh, but her leaf shall be green; and shall not be careful in the year of drought, neither shall cease from yielding fruit."

People who have their trust in mankind start to doubt whenever challenging times come. Our trust should be in God, so when hard times come, we will not doubt, but have supernatural strength to persevere.

When worry clouds our lives, we should "worry or meditate" on the Word of God. We should think about it all the time by focusing on the Word of God just like we do when we worry. Then, instead of stress, we would have peace because we'd be renewing our mind.

4. Renewing your mind makes you wiser.

Psalms 119:97-100

"O' how I love thy law! It is my meditation all the day. Thou through thy commandments hast made me wiser than mine enemies: for they are ever with me. I have more understanding than all my teachers: for thy testimonies are my meditations. I understand more than the ancients, because I keep thy precepts."

Even a cow can show us how to renew our mind. Whenever a cow lays down to rest, it chews its cud. The cow has several stomachs and is constantly chewing its food over and over again to get the most out of it. That is how we should be with the Word of God; we need to go over it again and again.

If you do not have tenacity concerning your dream or promise from the Lord, someone will try to come and take it from you. Take this example from a chicken. When a chicken is sitting on her eggs, the chicken will fight you if you ever try to get close to her eggs. We should be like the sitting hen, willing to fight rather than be pulled away from the Word of God.

5. Renewing your mind enriches your life.

Proverbs 4:20-24

"My son, attend to my words; incline thine ear unto my sayings. Let them not depart from thine eyes; keep them in the midst of thine heart. For they are life unto those that find them, and health to all their flesh. Keep thy heart with all diligence; for out of it are the issues of life. Put away from thee a froward mouth, and perverse lips put far from thee."

12

I Want My Daddy

This is the cry of boys and girls, men and women all over the world! If the enemy can destroy the relationship that was created to be a blueprint of what our relationship should look like with our spiritual father, God our Father, many will leave the earth not producing what is inside of them!

Malachi 4:4–6

Remember the law of my servant Moses, the decrees and laws I gave him at Horeb for all Israel. See, I will send you the prophet Elijah before that great and dreadful day of the LORD comes. He will turn the hearts of the fathers to their children, and the hearts of the children to their fathers; or else I will come and strike the land with a curse. (NIV)

As I sat in my counseling session, my counselor asked me about my childhood. I burst into tears. I didn't really know where to start; but I had been praying and asking God, *"Why can't I maintain healthy relationships with men and sometimes women?"* It seemed like I would always end up getting hurt or hurting someone. How far could I trace the beginning of this open door? I remember as far back as sixth grade; guys always left me for someone else. I thought, *"Am I not good enough, pretty enough, educated enough? What is the problem? Where did this curse come from?"*

After much prayer even more was revealed. Part of the answer came where this first started. The enemy looks for a road, which is a thought that he can continually drive to determine the outcome of your life. One of my dad's sisters and I were talking about something else on the phone in 2012 at the beginning of the year, but the conversation turned and she thought through the Holy Spirit, that it was necessary that she share something with me that I never knew.

My parents separated when I was about two years old. One day my dad was scheduled to pick me up and I was going with them to Orange, Texas. My Aunt Florence said that my Aunt Maurine, who had recently passed late in 2010, told her that my dad picked me up and once they put me in the car at two years old, I cried all the way to Orange, Texas, and cried all the way back to Houston, Texas. I cried because I didn't want my dad to drop me back off and continue to be separated from him. I loved my dad so much. I just wanted to sit in his lap. I wanted him to read me bed time stories, and let me know what to look for in relationships, etc. But when he and my mother separated, through that separation, there was a path set to literally destroy my life.

The spirit of abandonment, rejection, low self esteem and poverty haunted me all of my life. I was looking for love in all the wrong places. It wasn't that my dad didn't love me and my brothers but he and my mom couldn't resolve the issue that drove them apart. The enemy wanted his voice silenced in our life as we grew up. I needed my daddy. God was calling me in to preparation even back as far as I can remember. God was preparing me for right now to share with people all over the world. He was using all of this to bring me to realize I am Created 2 Produce. What the enemy meant for bad God worked it for my good. He is doing the same for you. God needs families to escape to a safe place with their children until the proper time to come out. This is what Mary and Joseph did. Until the enemy that was set to destroy their family was actually dead.

This is the same spirit that Herod issued in the bible to kill all of the male seed at the age of two years old and under. The Gospel according to St. Matthew, says that King Herod ordered baby boys to be killed, for fear that one of them would grow up to usurp his throne. According to this Gospel, Jesus and his parents escaped to Egypt, returning only after Herod's death. I don't look at this as only natural gender – but any man or woman who has a call on their life, to destroy the works of the enemy. Satan wants them dead at an early age.

The enemy sought to kill my father's seed at an early age. My father was shifted out of our home because the enemy didn't want our family to be a voice in the earth to restore families. He feared that we would produce too many seeds in the earth and alter his plans to destroy the family.

But I come with all power in me to help as many families as possible, so they will not experience the principalities and powers that rule in darkness over the family. This is the first institution that God created. I hate the devil and what he has done to all who have been victims of broken homes. I will do as many workshops, seminars, training and equipping in this area, with the help of other powerful ministries that have been called to this mountain.

The enemy wanted to kill my dad and he wanted my mother to be left alone from the very beginning, so that the purpose of God couldn't be revealed through our generation. Yes, absolutely, the first command God gave to mankind was to "be fruitful and multiply." Genesis 1:28: Then God blessed them and said, "Be fruitful and multiply. Fill the earth and govern it. Reign over the fish in the sea, the birds in the sky, and all the animals that scurry along the ground."

Deuteronomy 7:14: You shall be blessed above all people; there shall not be a male or female barren among you or among your livestock.

Exodus 23:26: There shall be no one miscarrying or barren in your land; I will fulfill the number of your days.

What happens when the male and female can't come together? There is no birthing. Many are deceived to think it's about you not getting along with that person that God has joined you with for such a time as this. Beware of the wiles of the enemy. He comes to steal, kill and destroy. But Christ has come that you might have life. I speak life into every dead family, those who have not only died but have been buried; many relationships will be restored according to the Word of God.

I have a call on my life to share with as many people as possible, if at all possible keep your family together. Ultimately it's about the destiny of God being or not being revealed in the earth through you.

On the day that my dad picked me up, I cried for hours because I didn't want him to leave me. I couldn't even enjoy the time I had with him for thinking about what would happen when I got home. It left a road or a path for other male and female relationships of fear or a longing.

I remember during my high school days when I met this guy who was assigned to me to tempt me into having sex for the first time. He was showing me what I thought was love, but it was pure lust sent to destroy my life.

Of course, I didn't do like Joseph did when he was tempted by the king's wife; I didn't flee. I didn't run from him, but ran into his arms. This was one of the worst mistakes of my life. I began to cut class, leave school and sleep with him continually.

I disobeyed my mom (the wages of sin is death) until one month, I realized that I was pregnant as a teenager. I didn't know what to do; I was so afraid. I didn't tell anyone but my best friend Veronica. We were too young to even know how to handle the situation. I know I was about three months pregnant and still praying for my cycle to come every day. I didn't want to be in CPS with Naomi Hilliard (you would have to know my mom to understand that statement).

At that time, I was a majorette in high school, and we had to go to summer camp. I remember praying that my cycle would come. One day we were at camp and it started raining really hard. We had to run a long way to get back to our room from training. Once we got to the room, I went to the restroom and I thought I had started my cycle, I told my best friend Veronica and we jumped and shouted saying, "Thank You Jesus, Hallelujah!"

We went to Astroworld later that night. We rode every high and low ride there was before leaving. I started to feel really bad. I thought I started my cycle but once I got home the blood was coming in such a strong force I realized that I was hemorrhaging.

I had to ask my mom to come to the rest room because I was in so much pain. I was in the worst pain of my life and blood was everywhere. She asked me "San, have you ever had sex?"

I looked in her eyes and said, "No." I was too scared to tell her the truth. She took me to the doctor, because I almost hemorrhaged to death. It was beyond belief. I lost my baby that night while sitting in the restroom. I still wasn't truly aware of the danger I was in. When we got there the doctor told my mom I had a miscarriage. She had to put me in the hospital for almost a week and told me to tell no one.

Of course I told the guy, and when I did, our relationship took a u-turn. He left me hook line and sinker. I cried beyond belief; I just wanted to be loved. I wanted to be accepted and thought because I gave myself to him that he loved me. It was a lie sent from the pit of hell. It was pure lust. I truly thank God that I didn't have to go through being a young single teen age mother at a very early age in my life.

I ended up in and out of different relationships with men, in adultery and fornication. It was a strategy from the pit of hell to alter my turning points in life.

After much counsel with my counselor, I realized I needed to deal with these points in my life, and go back and close some doors that had allowed other major events to almost alter my life.

There is a set time for every season under the sun – for all that you have been through – the time was set – let it be! Something good is going to come from this!

Ecclesiastes 3 (NIV):

A Time for Everything

There is a time for everything, and a season for every activity under the heavens:

> ² a time to be born and a time to die,
> a time to plant and a time to uproot,
> ³ a time to kill and a time to heal,
> a time to tear down and a time to build,
> ⁴ a time to weep and a time to laugh,
> a time to mourn and a time to dance,
> ⁵ a time to scatter stones and a time to gather them,
> a time to embrace and a time to refrain from embracing,
> ⁶ a time to search and a time to give up,
> a time to keep and a time to throw away,
> ⁷ a time to tear and a time to mend,
> a time to be silent and a time to speak,

> ⁸ a time to love and a time to hate,
> a time for war and a time for peace.

A Set Time With Daddy

The set time has now come for my relationship to be restored with my father. For over ten years now my relationship with my father has been restored. The most profound words he said to me in my darkest hour were, "San whatever you do, don't ever stop serving God." He said things like, "San, watch how people act naturally; it is an indication where their spiritual relationship is with God. He reminded me when he and my mom separated how he stopped serving God and got on the wrong road. Even though I didn't get to spend a lot of time with him as a young girl, God knew He would allow a time that the scripture would be fulfilled. He is with me every step of the way now covering me as a father should. I love my daddy with all of my heart.

I decree and declare every male or female that grew up without a father all those years will be restored, and I decree and declare the relationship with your father will be restored. The Word of God declares according to Malachi 4, the curse is broken!

Not only will your relationship with your natural father be restored, but the relationship with your spiritual Father shall be restored as well. You have been suffering long enough. This is your turning point, forgive and be restored in Jesus Name. I pray you will be like the sons of Issachar, who could discern the signs of the times and knew what to do in each season.

You are Created 2 Produce!

I am sent in this day to be a midwife, helping those who are pregnant with purpose to deliver and bring forth their miracle assigned from the Kingdom of God. As it is in Heaven regarding you, I decree you will be used to manifest it in the earth for such a time as this.

Turning Point - Fathers Needing Turned Hearts

What does it mean for a father to turn his heart toward his child? Well, what is the opposite of having a heart turned toward a child? The opposite is to have the heart turned away. Here are three examples:

Fathers, you can have your heart turned away from your children simply by ignoring them – by being so swallowed up in your work that all they get are the dregs of your life.

You can have your heart turned away from your children by being abusive. It may be that without even hearing yourself your communication with them is a litany of disapproval and put-downs. Why? Because your heart is not toward them. You don't feel what they feel. Your heart is frozen in a posture of habitual unkindness. Or worse in our day is the increase (or increasingly revealed) sexual abuse of children. And where, then, is the father's heart? It is curled around like a snake in love with its own tail and consuming itself on its own filthy passions.

Or you can have your heart turned away from your children through an embittered spirit of disappointment: that you are forgotten by them, or that they have let you down in the way they live, or that they have taken you for granted and never said thanks for all you did. Where is the heart then? In the poisoned puddle of self-pity that threatens to grow into an ocean of resentment.

Turning Point - Children Needing Turned Hearts

What about the other way around? What about children with hearts that need to be turned toward their fathers and mothers? What kind of hearts would this apply to today?

It would apply to rebellious and disobedient children. It could be a five year old or a fifteen year old. Where is the heart? It sits in front of the mirror of the soul trying to convince itself that the witch-face of cockiness and independence is really the fairest face in the land.

Turning Point - God's Word To Parents And Children

Notice, it does not say that any father or child can turn the heart of the other. That is not your responsibility. But your own heart is. So the word of God to fathers (and mothers!) today is this:

- Turn your hearts to your children:
- Don't give them the dregs of your life.
- Turn your hearts to your children:
- Don't be unkind,
- Don't constantly criticize,

- Don't even think the wicked thoughts that lead to sexual abuse.
- Turn your hearts toward your children:
- Let the bitterness go, at least from your side forgive, and roll the burden onto God.
- And the word to children is this:
- Turn your hearts toward your father (and mother!)
- Don't rebel; obey!
- Turn your hearts toward your fathers and mothers and grandparents:
- Don't forget them or neglect them; care for them.
- Turn your hearts toward your father:

The road to restoration may be as long as life. It may involve extensive counseling with a wise Christian therapist. But in your heart the decisive step can be taken, and must be taken. The feeling of having been victimized must cease to justify animosity.

Time to be Revealed

As with physical birth, there is a set time for your spiritual baby to be revealed. The Word of God gives us insight to the concept of being revealed as sons and daughters of the Most High God.

You should keep in mind that:

1. You are revealed by name when God is with you.

Matthew 1:23

"Behold, the virgin shall be with child, and bear a Son, and they shall call His name Immanuel," which is translated, "God with us."

2. You are revealed when the Word of God in you begins to become flesh.

John 1:1-2, 14

In the beginning was the Word, and the Word was with God, and the Word was God. He was in the beginning with God...And the Word became flesh and dwelt among us, and we beheld His glory, the glory as of the only begotten of the Father, full of grace and truth.

3. You are revealed as you become one with the purpose of the Father and His Son, Jesus Christ.

John 10:30

"I [Jesus] and My Father are one."

    Joseph was one such man of God who realized His purpose in being revealed. Joseph revealed himself to his brothers after the painful turmoil of being left for dead by them and sold off into slavery for many of his young adult years in life. But Joseph had an "emotional revelation." The bible says that then Joseph could not restrain himself before all those who stood by him, and he cried out, "Make everyone go out from me!" So no one stood with him while Joseph made himself known to his brothers. And he wept aloud, and the Egyptians and the house of Pharaoh heard it. Then Joseph said to his brothers, "I am Joseph; does my father still live?" But his brothers could not answer him, for they were dismayed in his presence.

Because of the punishment they anticipated, the great emotion of Joseph, his manner of revelation, and the total shock of learning Joseph was not only alive but right in front of them, the brothers were dismayed. The ancient Hebrew word for dismayed (bahal) actually means, "amazed" or "frightened" or even "terrified."

"Come near to me" in Genesis 45:4 implies the brothers cringed back in terror. Jewish legends say the brothers were so shocked that their souls left their bodies and it was only by a miracle of God their souls came back.

Joseph's testimony: And Joseph said to his brothers, "Please come near to me." So they came near. Then he said: "I am Joseph your brother, whom you sold into Egypt. But now, do not therefore be grieved or angry with yourselves because you sold me here; for God sent me before you to preserve life. For these two years the famine has been in the land, and there are still five years in which there will be neither plowing nor harvesting. And God sent me before you to preserve posterity for you in the earth, and to save your lives by a great deliverance. So now it was not you who sent me here, but God; and He has made me a father to Pharaoh, and lord of his entire house, and a ruler throughout all the land of Egypt.

My point is, after all you went through, the enemy would have thought you would be left for dead, but you can't die it's not your time. You have much to do in this world to bring many out of bondage. The enemy is going to be shocked that you made it because God would have worked on your character and integrity. You will tell all, *"you meant it to kill me; but God is a deliverer."*

Many people thought I would have never made it through all of the challenges I went through, but guess what? I'm still here. On purpose. Chosen for such a time as this. To bring many out to their turning points.

13

Let It Be

Who hasn't wanted to ask in the face of a life-altering change, "How can this be?" I want to conclude reflecting on Mary's miracle.

Holy confusion is a natural part of the life of any believer; indeed, any person. Ironically, earlier in Luke's Gospel, Zechariah, the soon-to-be father of John the Baptist, doesn't fare as well with his question. When he doubts that his elderly wife will conceive a son, a manifestly testy angel strikes him dumb. When Mary airs her confusion, the angel politely furnishes her with an explanation albeit a confusing one. In my opinion, it's a striking example of biblical favoritism for women.

God will confirm what He has put inside of you. It will be like fire shut up in your bones. I use to sneak to churches, women conferences and home prayer meetings with men and women who dared to pray and preach the Word of God with power. Back then churches were being birthed in shopping strips. I would go in and be drenched with the power of the Holy Ghost. It wasn't popular and kind of taboo. But I wanted something more; it wasn't really me it was the Holy Spirit leading me to be open to receive this new thing in my life.

When I would hear these powerful men and women of God I would cry, dance, leap and shout. One thing I couldn't deny was the Power of God. It was like I was getting a fix. I don't mean to offend the church people but the kingdom of God needs a fix from the Holy Ghost that will change your life.

I thought, *Oh my God! I want to have the presence of God work like that in me.* I gleaned, bought tapes, CDs, sowed seed in their ministries, and I would listen to them preach all night long. I would put my plugs in my ear and tears would fall everywhere. The sound, the sound, the deep was calling me. It was like a satisfaction that I never felt before.

When God started letting me know what He wanted me to do in life, I thought like Mary, *How can this be?* No one will believe me. I don't have the help. I don't have the education. I don't preach like them or pray like him…Geez! I sounded like Moses handing out all of my human excuses.

Don't you know that God already knows what is wrong with you?

My family was diametrically opposed to that saying. He told me just like He told Mary, "The Holy Spirit will overshadow you." I finally said, "Let it be."

Each time I did anything for God publically or privately, He showed up. When I witnessed on the street, taught in shelters, in church, prayer meetings, or ministered in song, the Holy Spirit always showed up. He assured me that He would. It was amazing every time He did. He used me to draw others to Him. Jeremiah 1:5. "Before I formed you in the womb I knew you

LET IT BE

(Cassandra), before you were born I set you (Cassandra) apart; I appointed you (Cassandra) as a prophet to the nations."

I stand amazed!

God asked me this: "Are you going to believe the Word or not? Are you going to let people that don't know anything about what I appointed you to do stop you?"

I submit to you that you not doubt what God has put inside you. It has been placed inside of you by God. He knows the plans He has for you. It has already been prepared. It's not anything just recently thought about or that He just thought about today. It has already been prophesied and it has already been foretold.

Look at the pattern God gives us in the word of the birth of Jesus! Look at the people that He uses to bring the Messiah into the earth and don't second guess your call again. God can call you wherever you are. Just like He did with me, the girl who came straight out of Kashmere Garden, Houston, Texas, 8714 Spaulding, from in a single family home on welfare and I was the least likely to be chosen.

Just like He did with me, He can use you to change a nation. God's got this! Go with the flow! Stop resisting, it's going to be alright and that's His promise to you!

Don't be as the men and women of today who fail to keep their promises. God was faithful to all of us. He kept His promise that Jesus would be born into this world. Joseph was faithful to God and married Mary and kept her a virgin. The scriptures said that a virgin would give birth. If Joseph had had sex before she gave birth, that promise of God would not have been true. God has been and is faithful. He is an example of faithfulness and He calls us to be faithful. What do you do when the people closest to you do not understand that what you have conceived is spiritual and not natural? Before you were created in your mother's womb, God had already planned how you would manifest what you are carrying to deliver to a certain group of people.

I grew up in the Baptist church during a time when it was not popular for a woman to announce that she had been called to minister the Word of God. How many of you have grown up in a place where what God put in you would not be received? It goes against everything. Many family members and friends have walked off from people who were just trying to do what God called them to do.

I am reminded of Joseph, and how he couldn't handle that his fiancé was pregnant before he even touched her, and how he would be her husband, and she was pregnant with something that had nothing to do with him. He was so confused, this baby wouldn't look like him, talk like him or act like him. How many men and women are faced with this same challenge? The one person that you love so much, announces to you, "I'm pregnant with destiny." The purpose of God is to start a ministry, a business, write a book, etc., and the one closest to you does not understand.

I remember when I was married, my ex-husband told me, "if you ever preach the word, I will divorce you." I was devastated, I couldn't help what God had given me, how would I handle this situation? I prayed and asked the Holy Spirit to help me in this, and He did. I was given wisdom by God, not by me, to just be his wife and not press the issue, and in the proper time, it would manifest. I'll never forget how he testified how God showed him who I was, the rest is history. I am so grateful to God that he accepted what God said. Most believers don't understand seed, time and then harvest.

It is a process and you are in the incubator of time. God is using every moment to prepare you for your purpose in life. There are many of you reading this book you have been trying to convince the people closest to you, about what God has shared with you about your calling or who you are. They don't understand you, sometimes if you tell the truth, you don't understand either. You need the Holy Ghost to visit them and put the matter in God's hand. Go and flee with someone who is pregnant at the same time you are, or have already been there and done that; Mary went and found Elizabeth, her cousin who confirmed what she was carrying. In this season God will connect you to people who celebrate you and not just tolerate you. This is your season to be acknowledged in the public, that which God announced to you privately.

If you will obey Him, God will let one person receive you and believe you and both of your babies will leap inside. Go ahead, start that business, start that ministry, start a home Bible study or prayer meeting with the help of spiritual authority, guiding you along the way. You shouldn't be out there alone, but your spiritual mother or father should validate who you are.

Have you ever been around people that make you get excited about what you haven't really shared with a lot of people?

It makes you free inside when you don't feel like you have to hold back or when you talk to them and they can relate to where you are.

I assure you today, God will handle it all and it will come to pass. God bless Joseph for hearing the voice of God in a dream to not put Mary away; that she indeed was telling the truth of what God said to her. He could have publicly humiliated her, but he was a righteous man of God and he covered her and the gift inside of her; even thou I know he didn't fully understand. God bless the men of God that will validate their wives and daughters naturally and spiritually, for what God has put inside of them, and will cover them in the transition and the great turning point of their lives.

He could have interrupted the plan of God. Have you ever wanted to put so much pressure on people, who say they have been visited by the very presence of God, in regards to who they are? And because you have authority over a situation, you could cause it to abort or live.

I'm reminded of Moses going to Pharaoh and saying to him, "God said, let my people go." Just think, he was responsible for people never living out destiny and if God wouldn't have raised up a Moses to speak up for them, they would have died in slavery or the wilderness! I say today for you, "Let my brother and sister go you spirit of Pharaoh." Be free today in Jesus Name!

Go ahead and stop procrastinating and just say, "Let it be," even though you don't understand what God is doing in your natural mind. "Let it be according to Your Word, oh God."

1 Corinthians 2:9 says, "However, as it is written: "No eye has seen, no ear has heard, no mind has conceived what God has prepared for those who love him."

I leave every reader with these words. Once you let go, get out of the way and let God, you will experience the greatest turning point in your life. Just do like Mary and say, "Let It Be According To Your Word." God will take care of the rest. You will not be able to imagine what God has next for you. Remember you are Created 2 Produce!

SOURCES:

*David M. Fergusson, John Horwood and Michael T. Lynsky, "Parental Separation, Adolescent Psychopathology, and Problem Behaviors," Journal of the American Academy of Child and Adolescent Psychiatry 33 (1944).

**Denise B. Kandel, Emily Rosenbaum and Kevin Chen, "Impact of Maternal Drug Use and Life Experiences on Preadolescent Children Born to Teenage Mothers," Journal of Marriage and the Family56 (1994).

***Alfred A. Messer, "Boys Father Hunger: The Missing Father Syndrome," Medical Aspects of Human Sexuality, January 1989.

****F. Furstenberg, A. Cherlin, Divided Families . Harvard Univ. Press. 1991.

*****Christian Apologetics & Research Ministry. "What is meant when it says man is made in the image of God?" Article found at: http://carm.org/questions/about-people/what-meant-when-it-says-man-made-image-god

BIO

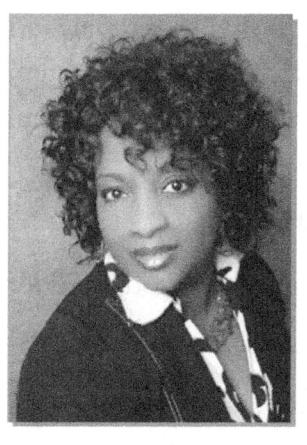

Dr. Cassandra E. Scott (a.k.a. Pastor C) is completely committed to restoring the people of God's faith, families, finances, and futures. She founded Created 2 Produce, Cassandra Scott Ministries and Turning Point Faith with a desire to help people find their turning point to destiny.

Pastor C is humbled by her God-given gifts of teaching, preaching, pastoring, and evangelizing. Yet she delivers in a powerful way in her weekly speaking engagements, bible studies, one-on-one mentoring, planned conferences, training, and workshops.

Cassandra was told by doctors that she could not have children, but by the grace of God, today she is a dedicated mother of two beautiful daughters: Garelyn Evett and Gabrielle Chrishelle, and a handsome son, Gary Emerson II. She uses her gift to help other women having difficulties conceiving to bring forth children. God also gifted her as a spiritual midwife giving birth to a number of pastors & leaders. An anointed teacher and student of the Word, Pastor C earned her Doctorate, Masters, & Bachelors in Theology at Immanuel Temple School accredited through Calvary Theological Seminary/Cornerstone University of Lake Charles, LA under the leadership of Dr. Barbara Wright, President/Founder.

Cassandra believes that empowerment is both a spiritual and physical matter, so she empowers people financially through business opportunities every chance she gets. She has several business & ministry venues, some of which are:

- **Turning Point Faith Ministries (TPF)**

    Church congregation founded by Cassandra Scott in 2008.

- **Cassandra Scott Ministries/Created 2 Produce (C2P)**

    Personal ministry platform; training, one-on-one mentorship, speaking, and conferences.

- **C.H.A.R.M., Inc.**

    Cassandra's House of Angels Residential Manor, a planned facility for women & girls.

- **Independent Beauty Consultant - Future Executive Sr. Sales Director, Mary Kay**

    A successful director with Mary Kay establishing leader consultants across the nation.

- **Ignite Independent Business Associate**

    Helping non-profits increase their organization's funding through Stream Energy.

Made in the USA
Monee, IL
10 August 2024

63038367R00095